15 MINUTE MEALS

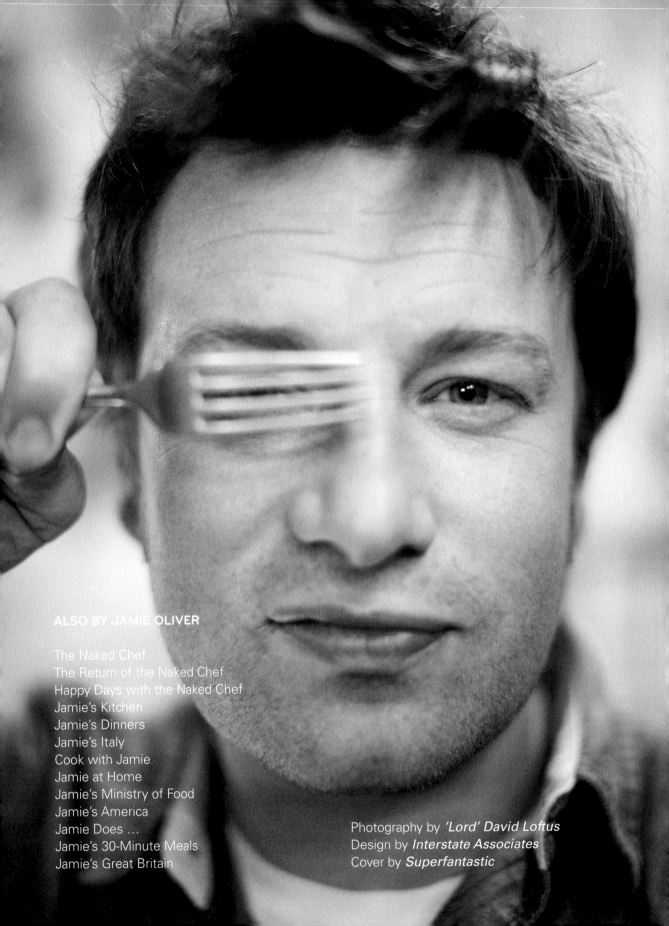

ALSO BY JAMIE OLIVER

Photography by *'Lord' David Loftus*
Design by *Interstate Associates*
Cover by *Superfantastic*

15 MINUTE MEALS

MICHAEL JOSEPH

an imprint of

PENGUIN BOOKS

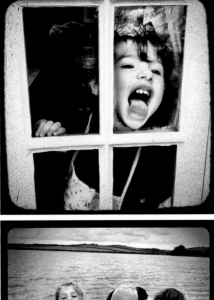 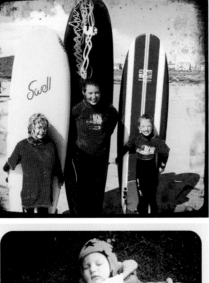 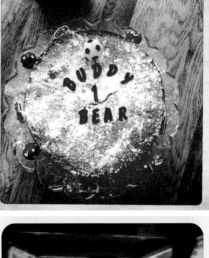

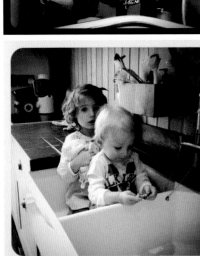 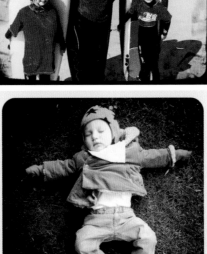 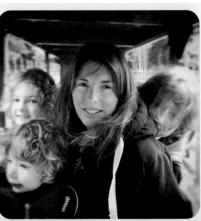

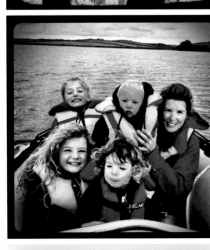 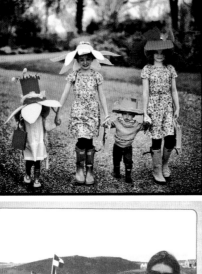 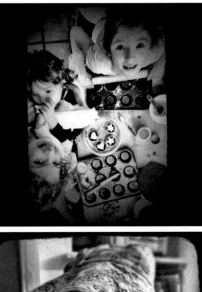

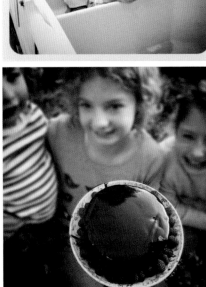 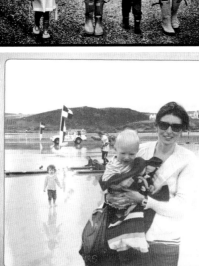 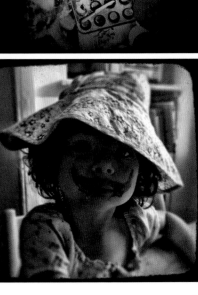

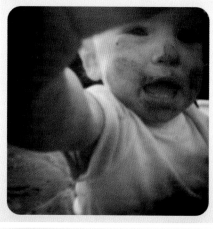

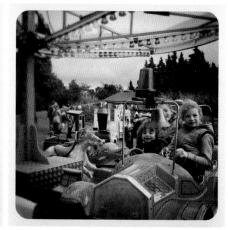

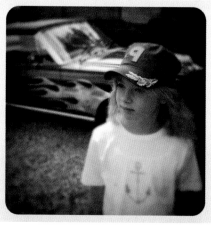

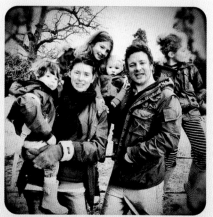

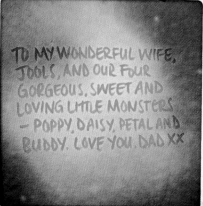

TO MY WONDERFUL WIFE,
JOOLS, AND OUR FOUR
GORGEOUS, SWEET AND
LOVING LITTLE MONSTERS
— POPPY, DAISY, PETAL AND
BUDDY. LOVE YOU. DAD XX

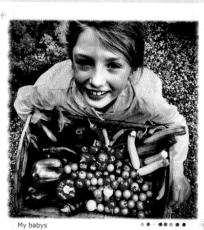

My babys

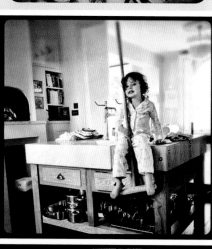

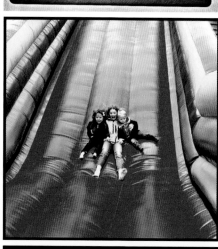

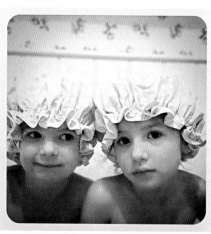

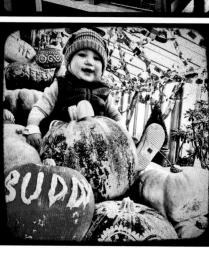

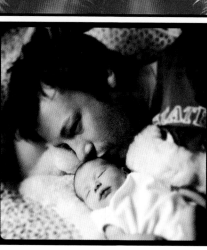

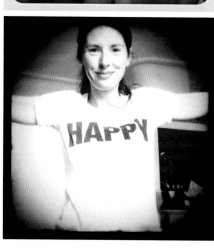

MICHAEL JOSEPH

Published by the Penguin Group

Penguin Books Ltd
80 Strand,
London WC2R 0RL, England

Penguin Group (USA) Inc.
375 Hudson Street,
New York, New York 10014, USA

Penguin Group (Canada)
90 Eglinton Avenue East, Suite 700,
Toronto, Ontario, Canada M4P 2Y3
(a division of Pearson Penguin Canada Inc.)

Penguin Ireland
25 St Stephen's Green,
Dublin 2, Ireland
(a division of Penguin Books Ltd)

Penguin Group (Australia)
250 Camberwell Road,
Camberwell, Victoria 3124, Australia
(a division of Pearson Australia Group Pty Ltd)

Penguin Books India Pvt Ltd
11 Community Centre,
Panchsheel Park, New Delhi – 110 017, India

Penguin Group (NZ)
67 Apollo Drive,
Rosedale, Auckland 0632, New Zealand
(a division of Pearson New Zealand Ltd)

Penguin Books (South Africa) (Pty) Ltd
Block D, Rosebank Office Park,
181 Jan Smuts Avenue, Parktown North,
Gauteng 2193, South Africa

Penguin Books Ltd, Registered Offices:
80 Strand, London WC2R 0RL, England

www.penguin.com
www.jamieoliver.com

First published 2012
001

Copyright © Jamie Oliver, 2012
Photography copyright © David Loftus, 2012

The moral right of the author has been asserted

Printed in Germany by Mohn media
Colour reproduction by Altaimage Ltd

A CIP catalogue record for this book
is available from the British Library

ISBN: 978–0–718–15780–7

SIMPLE

I'M SO EXCITED THAT YOU'RE STEPPING INTO THE WORLD OF *15-MINUTE MEALS*. THE PROMISE OF THIS BOOK IS SIMPLE: DELICIOUS, NUTRITIOUS, SUPER-FAST FOOD THAT'S A TOTAL JOY TO EAT AND PERFECT FOR BUSY PEOPLE LIKE YOU AND ME.

MY RELATIONSHIP WITH YOU, THE PUBLIC, AND THESE COOKBOOKS I WRITE IS AN INCREDIBLY IMPORTANT ONE. OVER 30 MILLION OF YOU HAVE BOUGHT MY BOOKS IN THE LAST 10 YEARS, AND I NEVER TAKE THAT AMAZING SUPPORT FOR GRANTED. WITH EACH NEW BOOK I FEEL A MASSIVE RESPONSIBILITY TO PUSH MYSELF AND GIVE YOU SOMETHING I REALLY BELIEVE IN; SOMETHING I THINK YOU WILL LOVE, WITH RECIPES THAT DELIVER ON EVERY LEVEL, AND THIS BOOK IS NO EXCEPTION. IT'S HAD A CLEAR GAME PLAN RIGHT FROM THE START, BECAUSE NOT ONLY AM I RESPONDING TO WHAT YOU ARE ALL SCREAMING OUT FOR – TASTY, QUICK, AFFORDABLE FOOD – I'M DOING IT WITH RECIPES THAT ARE ANCHORED IN BALANCE AND NUTRITION. **THE CREATION OF THIS BOOK HAS BEEN A REAL GAME CHANGER FOR ME.**

There are a lot of days when speed is key, and that's where *15-Minute Meals* comes into play. This book is categorically a tool to make you cook really fast, delicious, fresh food, any day of the week. Of course, slow cooking old-school, authentic recipes is the heart and soul of any great home cook, but this book is an expression of big, exciting flavours, fast, for busy people.

NUTRITIOUS
TOTAL JOY TO EAT

Because I passionately wanted this to be a cookbook you can use every day of the week, and not just for special occasions, health and nutrition had to be at the heart of it. So I wrote and cooked every recipe with my incredible nutritionists, Laura Parr and her team, looking over my shoulder. They kept me on track, and kept a close eye on portion size, and as a result the recipes in this book are averaging about 580 calories per serving, which is great, so they'll fit easily into any main meal based on what we should be eating each day. It's really important to vary your recipe choices so that you feed your body with lots of different nutrients. Most importantly – because calories can be a useful but slightly blunt measure – keep in mind that these tasty meals are packed full of wholefoods, grains, veggies, fresh herbs, citrus, quality proteins and other beautiful things that will really help take care of you and your family.

Developing and writing the recipes, designing the pages, getting the timings right, and bringing the calories and nutrition to this happy place without compromising on flavour has all taken an awful lot of hard work. Every word, every sentence, has been debated, and every single stage of each recipe has been streamlined in order to give you these super-quick, tasty dishes. I can't tell you how hard it's been. I've had to be ruthless, rein myself in, and carefully weigh up every decision I've made, from the amount of ingredients I've used to the number of pans on the hob. But it's been totally worth it, because my food team and I are so excited about where we've finally got to with this book. So please trust in all the effort we've put in, and know that as long as you follow what I've written, and have the essential equipment that is vital for speed, you'll be enjoying these tasty, healthy meals in your own home, possibly even tonight.

I've taken inspiration from all over the world for these dishes, and they are undeniably delicious. But for me, the best thing of all is the fact that great flavours, unbelievable speed and nutritious, proper, everyday food can now come together in the same package.

Ultimately, *15-Minute Meals* is a frame of mind, and I think if you give it a proper go you'll really get into it. It's fun, dynamic, no-nonsense cooking. Yes, the first couple of times you cook a recipe it might take a little longer, but that's OK, it's not a race. There's a rhythm to these lovely recipes, and each has its own kind of beat. Once you embrace that and get into the spirit of the shortcuts and tips that I've given you, you'll definitely start knocking these meals out of the park in 15 minutes. And of course, it's not just about me as a chef being able to do it. These recipes have also been tested by cooks at all levels, from teenagers and OAPs to busy mums and dads, and their response has mirrored the excitement that my team and I have – so positive and enthusiastic. Every one of them has helped me navigate the recipes into the shape they're in today. If they can do it, so can you.

The food in this book is tasty, it's got attitude, and it's just as at home being served to a house full of students as it is by parents to their children.

I know there's a perception out there that real food costs much more to cook than fast food does, but that's a fallacy; the average cost of a tasty balanced meal in this book is about £3.80 per person – and that's using lovely, quality ingredients – which the majority of the time is way cheaper than an equivalent pre-packed meal, takeaway or bucket of junk food. And if you get your weekly shopping routine down, and get your head and cooking skills in the *15-Minute Meals* zone, it's even quicker than going out to pick up dinner from a drive-through. Of course pre-prepared food can have a useful place in your diet once in a while, I just passionately believe that this book can help empower and encourage people of all ages to want to make real food for themselves more often than not.

FAST

DELICIOUS

SO THERE YOU GO GUYS, THAT'S THE *15-MINUTE MEAL* PHILOSOPHY – FAST, TASTY, AFFORDABLE, GOOD-FOR-YOU FOOD. I GENUINELY HOPE YOU EMBRACE IT, BECAUSE I'M BUZZING ABOUT THIS IN SO MANY WAYS. IT'S ALL HERE FOR YOU, SO TAKE THE PHILOSOPHY ON BOARD AND RUN WITH IT. GOOD LUCK – I KNOW YOU CAN DO IT.

15

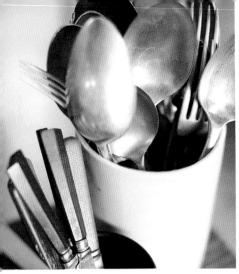
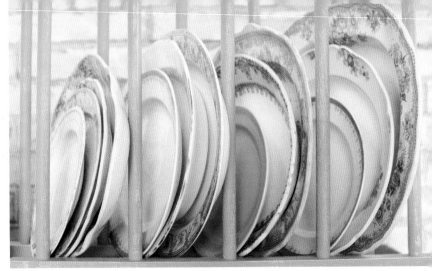
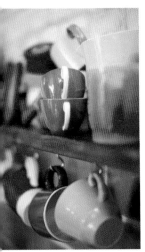

IMPORTANT HOW TO SERVE

Investing in a handful of large platters, boards and bowls is absolutely essential to the essence of *15-Minute Meals* – this is about family-service, sharing and getting amongst it. Ultimately the food is going to taste great whatever you serve it on, but if you're dishing up on random, average plates, you're totally missing the point. It doesn't have to be expensive – make your own boards with food-safe paint, like I do, or go to flea markets and pick up platters and bowls. Happy hunting.

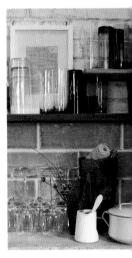
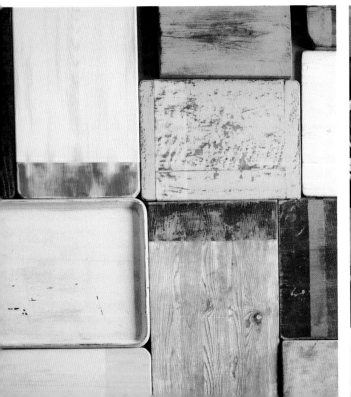
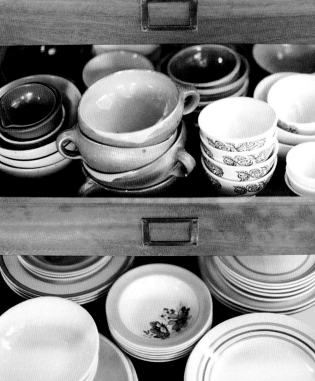

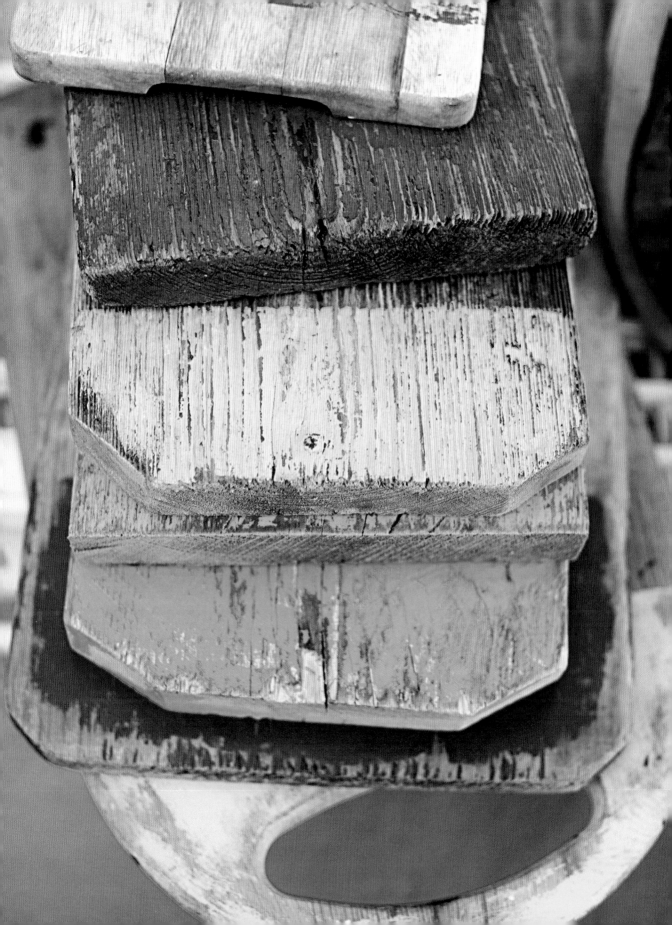

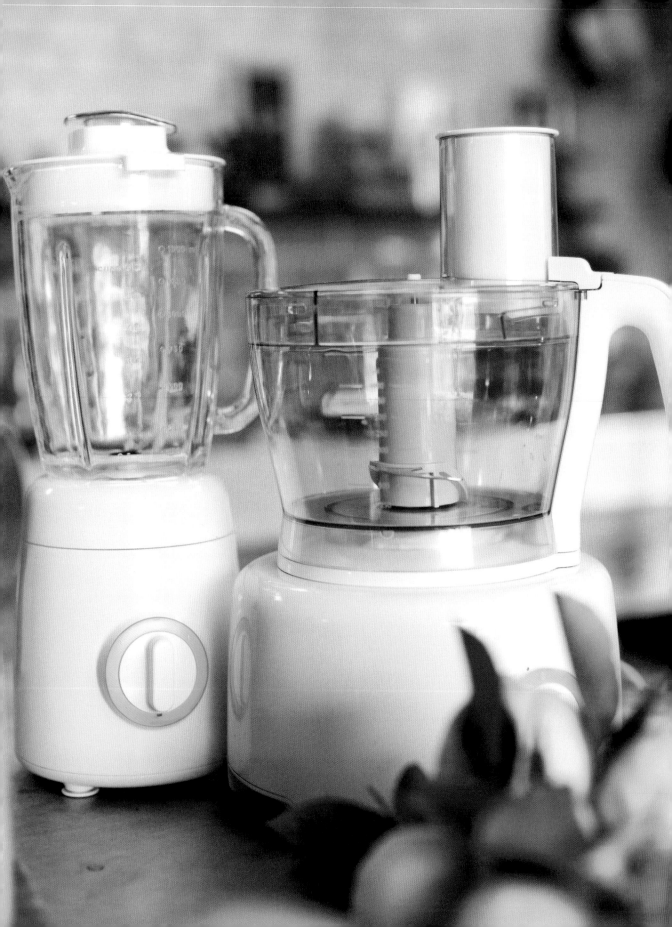

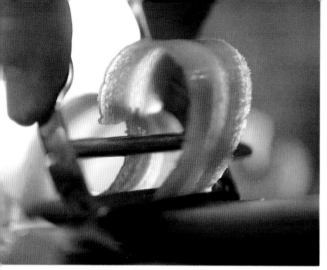

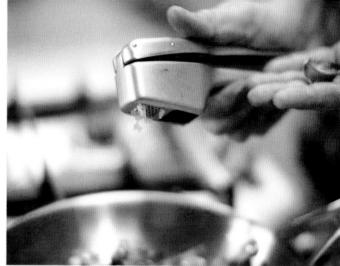

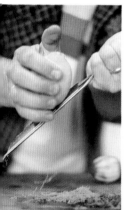

VERY IMPORTANT
HOW TO COOK FAST

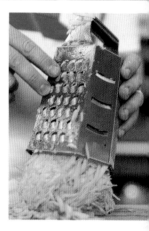

If you want to cook these tasty meals in 15 minutes, you must have these kitchen gadgets, utensils and bits of equipment. If you don't, you simply won't get the meals done in time. This is not a complex list, and to be frank, you can pick it all up super cheap these days if you want to (feel free to spend a bit more if you've got it). A food processor, liquidizer, stick blender and kettle are an absolute must – no compromise – they're essential. Good luck.

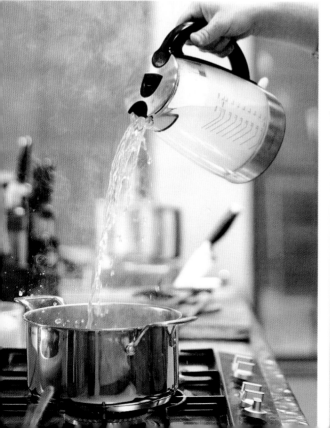

Equipment list

A good food processor	Pestle & mortar
Liquidizer	Garlic crusher
Stick blender	Tongs
Microwave	Fish slice
kettle	Wooden spoons
	Slotted spoon
Griddle pan	Spatula
Ovenproof frying pans	Potato masher
(roughly 30cm/25cm/20cm)	Speed-peeler
Lidded pans	
(roughly 25cm/20cm/15cm)	Box grater
2-level bamboo steamer	Fine grater
Large sturdy high-sided roasting trays	
Large non-stick baking trays	Measuring jug
	Measuring spoons
3 good-quality knives	Scales
(chef's/paring/bread)	Tin opener
Plastic chopping board	Rolling pin
Wooden chopping boards	Bottle opener
Mixing bowls	Large serving
Colander	platters, boards
Sieve	& bowls

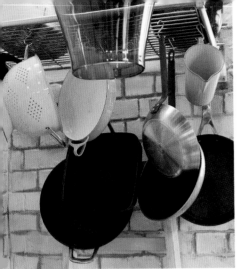
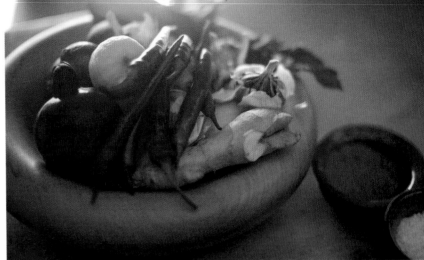

HOW TO OWN YOUR KITCHEN

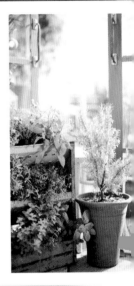

I've seen a lot of kitchens in my time, and bad organization is phenomenally common. It will hold you back in your cooking, so simply clear out the clutter and the random stuff like piggy banks and magazines that gather on surfaces but have nothing to do with food. It's common sense really: anything used for prep or stirring should be near to where you cook – everything around that area should be the kit you use most frequently, whether it's storage, knives, pans, even the fridge. This will allow you to be instinctive and fast in the kitchen. Happy spring clean.

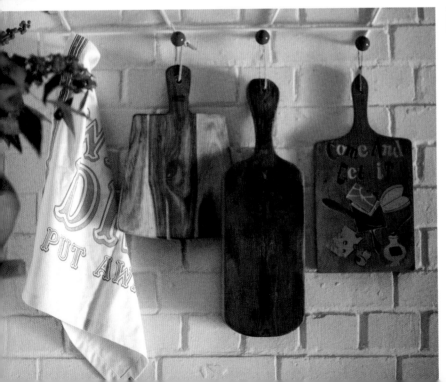
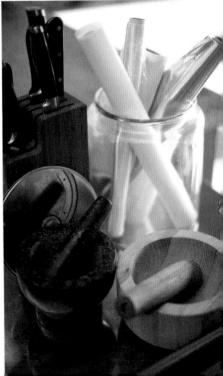

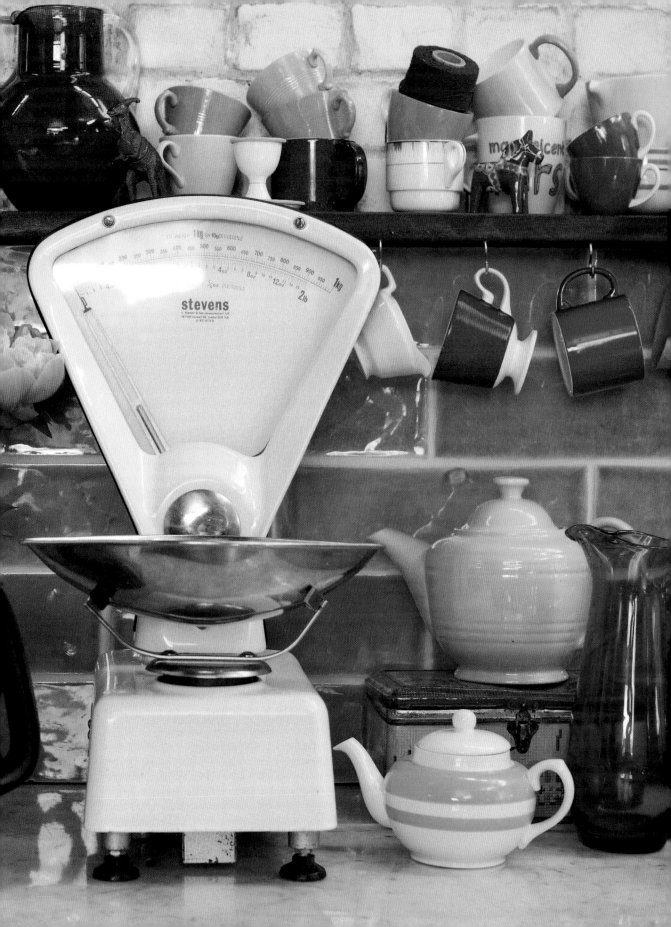

Pantry list

Baking: cocoa powder, cornflour, desiccated coconut, dried apricots, light brown sugar, plain flour, porridge oats, rose water, self-raising flour, vanilla paste

Dried herbs & spices: Cajun seasoning, caraway seeds, cayenne pepper, Chinese five-spice, cinnamon sticks, cumin seeds, curry leaves, dill, dried red chillies, English mustard powder, fennel seeds, fenugreek seeds, garam masala, ground allspice, ground cinnamon, ground cloves, ground coriander, ground ginger, kaffir lime leaves, mustard seeds, nutmeg, oregano, saffron, smoked chipotle or ancho chillies, smoked paprika, sweet smoked paprika, thyme, turmeric

Dried pasta & noodles: farfalle, fettucine, fusilli, linguine, macaroni, orecchiette, penne, shells, spaghetti, whole-wheat fusilli & spaghetti, egg noodles, thin rice noodles

Jams & spreads: blackberry jam, cranberry jam, peanut butter, runny honey

Jarred food: grated horseradish, passata, preserved lemons, red peppers, sun-dried tomatoes

Mustards: Dijon, English, wholegrain

Nuts & seeds: almonds, blanched hazelnuts, Brazil nuts, cashews, pine nuts, shelled peanuts, shelled pistachios, pumpkin seeds, sesame seeds, shelled walnuts, sunflower seeds

Oils: extra virgin olive, olive, rapeseed, sesame, truffle

Pastes: harissa, miso paste or powder, Patak's curry pastes (korma, rogan josh, tikka), sun-dried tomato tapenade, tomato purée

Pickled & jarred vegetables: cauliflower, cornichons, gherkins, ginger, jalapeño chillies, red cabbage

Rice, grains & pulses: basmati rice, bulgur wheat, couscous, fine cornmeal, quinoa, Uncle Ben's 10-minute wholegrain rice, Uncle Ben's cooked packs of brown & wild rice

Sauces: black bean, hoi sin, hot chilli, HP, Lingham's chilli, low-salt soy, mint, quality mayonnaise, sweet chilli, Tabasco, Teriyaki, tomato ketchup, Worcestershire

Tinned foods: anchovy fillets, chickpeas, chopped tomatoes, light coconut milk, mixed beans, pineapple chunks, red kidney beans, red split lentils, water chestnuts

Vinegars: balsamic, red wine, rice or white wine, sherry

Miscellaneous: chicken & vegetable stock cubes, green tea bags

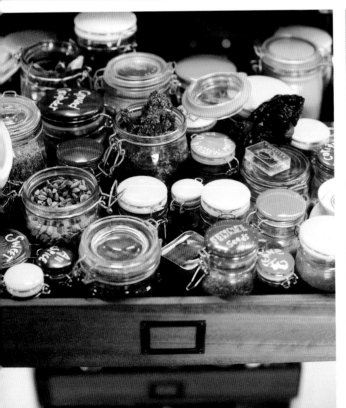

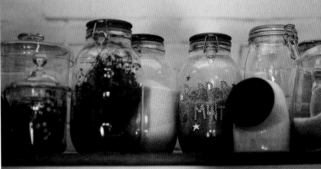

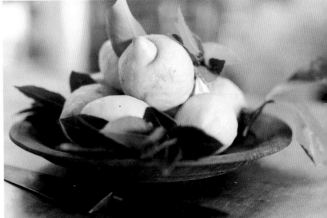

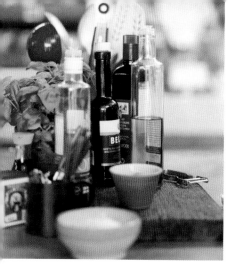

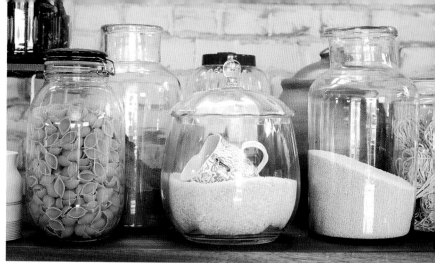

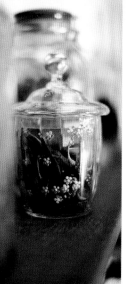

YOUR PANTRY

Here's my shopping list for a well-stocked pantry. These ingredients are really good flavour investments, and they pop up throughout the book. I love the fact that once you've stocked your shelves they're just ready, waiting for you to cook, so that they can brighten up your food. And they're nearly all non-perishable. If you want, go to *www.jamieoliver.com/15pantrylist* and you can get this list in an easy format that you can print out or view online, so that you can checklist what you need for next time you're shopping.

When it comes to fresh ingredients, if it's within your means, I strongly recommend supporting higher welfare and sustainable options for eggs, meat, fish, mayo, stock cubes, egg noodles and pasta. In return, this mindfulness will nearly always give you better flavour, and will make you feel better about your impact on the world.

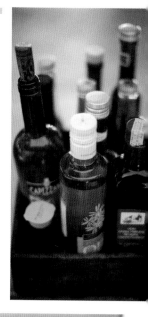

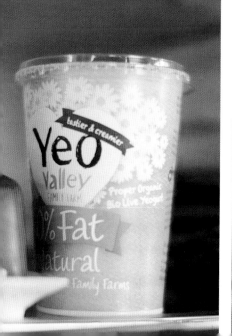

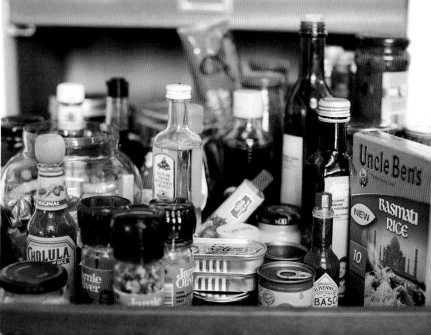

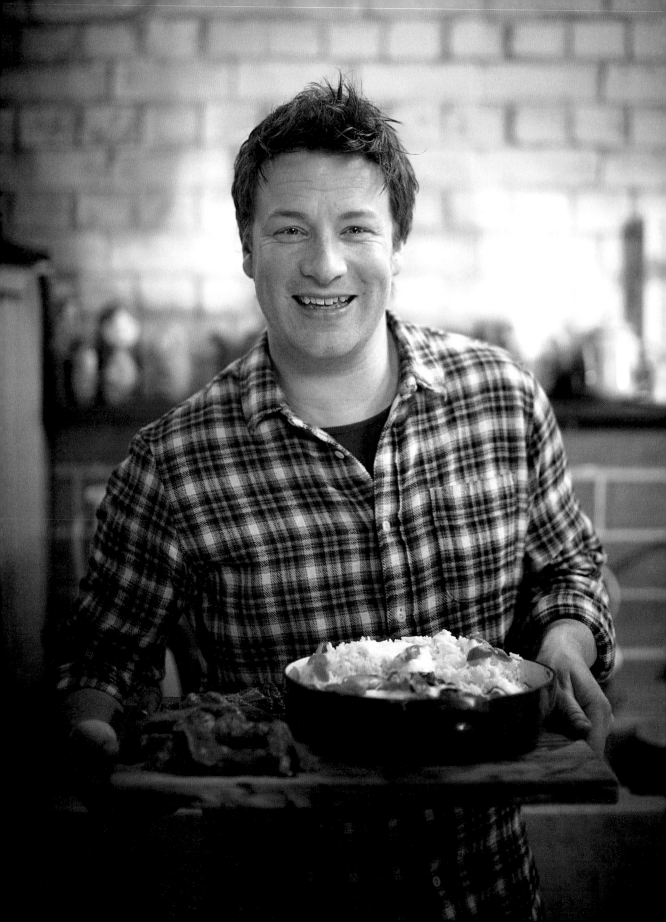

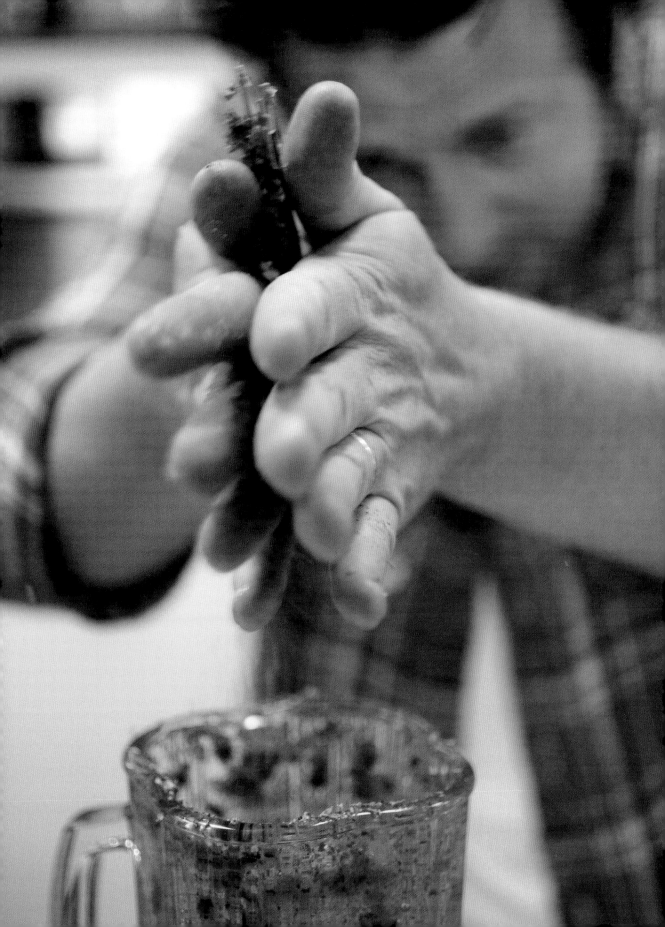

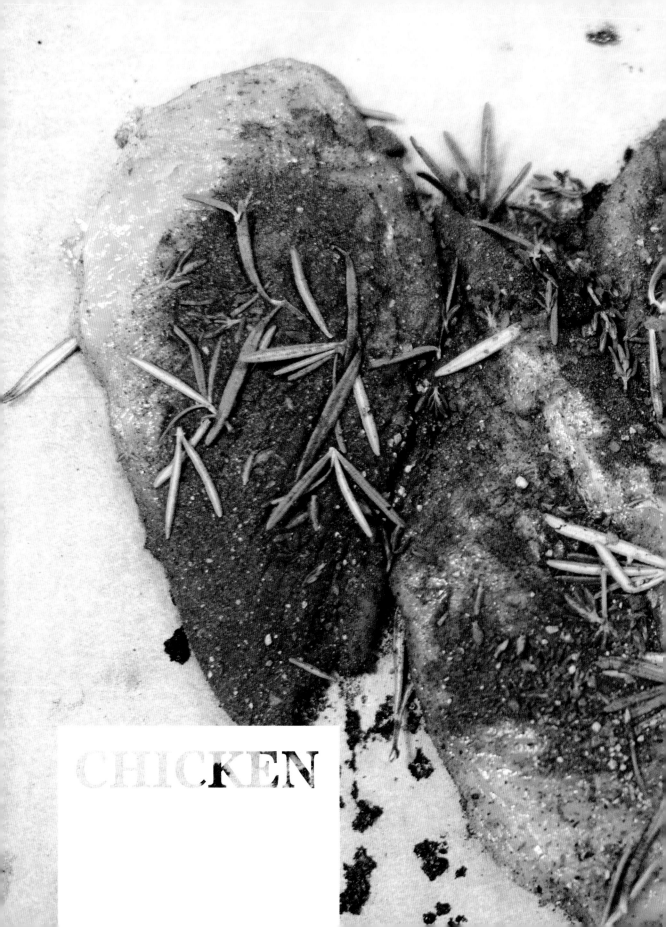

CHICKEN

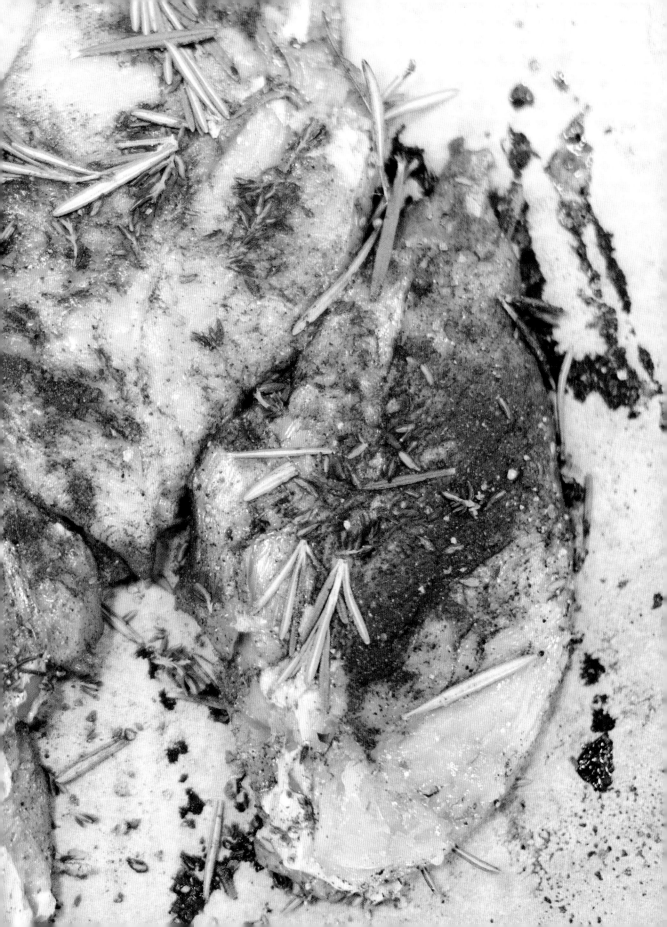

CHICKEN DIM SUM

COCONUT BUNS, CUCUMBER PICKLE & HOI SIN SAUCE

SERVES 4 | 795 CALORIES

Ingredients out • Kettle boiled • Food processor (bowl blade)
• 16 non-stick muffin cases • Two 25cm bamboo steamers
• Wok, medium-high heat • Small frying pan, low heat

Coconut buns

1 x 400g tin of light coconut milk
2 coconut milk tins (500g)
   of self-raising flour, plus extra
   for dusting

Chicken, pickles & garnishes

2 x 200g skinless chicken breasts
140g mixed mushrooms
3 tbsp hoi sin sauce, plus
   extra to serve
2 limes
200g tenderstem broccoli
1 cucumber
1 tbsp low-salt soy sauce
1 tbsp rice or white wine vinegar
½ a bunch of fresh coriander
3 tbsp sesame seeds
1 x 105g pack of pickled ginger
1–2 fresh red chillies

START COOKING

Pour the coconut milk into the processor with 2 heaped tins' worth of self-raising flour and a good pinch of salt, whiz to a dough, then tip on to a flour-dusted work surface • Roll the dough into a sausage shape, cut into 8 even-sized pieces, then place each one into a double-layered muffin case, and squeeze those into one layer of the steamer • Pour 5cm of boiling water into the wok, put the basket of buns on top with the lid on and leave to steam hard

Cut the chicken into 1cm strips and toss in a bowl with the roughly torn mushrooms, hoi sin sauce, juice of ½ a lime and a pinch of salt • Tip into the second steamer basket along with the trimmed broccoli and pop underneath the tray of buns for 5 minutes until cooked through • Speed-peel the cucumber into ribbons, toss in a bowl with the soy sauce, vinegar and a few torn coriander leaves, then with clean hands squeeze and scrunch everything together to make a pickle

Toast the sesame seeds in the frying pan until golden, then tip into a little bowl, cut the remaining 1½ limes into wedges, and serve with the pickled ginger and extra hoi sin sauce in little bowls • Serve the buns and chicken in the steamer trays, scattering everything with the remaining coriander leaves and finely sliced chilli

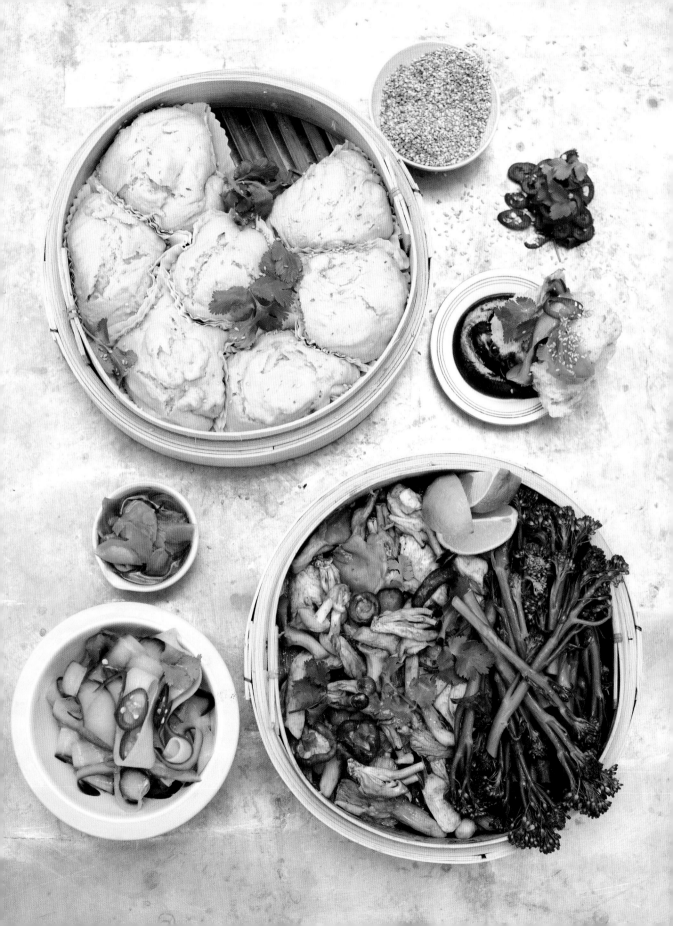

CHICKEN TIKKA
LENTIL, SPINACH & NAAN SALAD

SERVES 4 | 607 CALORIES

Ingredients out • *Griddle pan, high heat*
• *Small frying pan, medium-low heat* • *Liquidizer*

Chicken

2 x 200g skinless chicken breasts
2 heaped tsp Patak's tikka paste
4 chestnut mushrooms

Salad

4 spring onions
1 fresh red chilli
1 heaped tsp mustard seeds
½ tsp cumin seeds
olive oil
1 x 250g pack of ready-to-eat
  Puy lentils
1 ripe tomato
red wine vinegar
1 big bunch of fresh coriander
2 lemons
4 tbsp fat-free natural yoghurt
1 heaped tbsp cashew nuts
1 heaped tbsp mango chutney
1 tsp turmeric
2 naan breads
200g baby spinach
½ a cucumber
1 carrot
30g feta cheese

START COOKING

On a large sheet of greaseproof paper, toss the chicken with salt, pepper and the tikka paste • Fold over the paper, then bash and flatten the chicken to 1.5cm thick with a rolling pin • Place on the hot griddle pan with the halved mushrooms, turning after 3 or 4 minutes, until nicely charred and cooked through • Trim and finely slice the spring onions and half the chilli

Put the mustard and cumin seeds and 2 tablespoons of oil into the frying pan, followed by the sliced spring onion and chilli • Tip the lentils into the pan, squash in the tomato and add a pinch of salt and pepper and a splash of red wine vinegar • Toss occasionally for a couple of minutes, then turn the heat off • Rip the coriander stalks into the liquidizer with the juice of 1 lemon, the yoghurt, cashews, mango chutney and turmeric, then whiz up until smooth

Remove the cooked chicken and mushrooms from the griddle and put the naan on the pan • Tip the baby spinach on to a serving board or platter, scatter over the lentils, speed-peel the cucumber and carrot over the top and sprinkle over the mushrooms • Slice the chicken, naan and remaining chilli and arrange on top, then crumble over the feta and spoon over the dressing • Finish with the coriander leaves and serve with lemon wedges

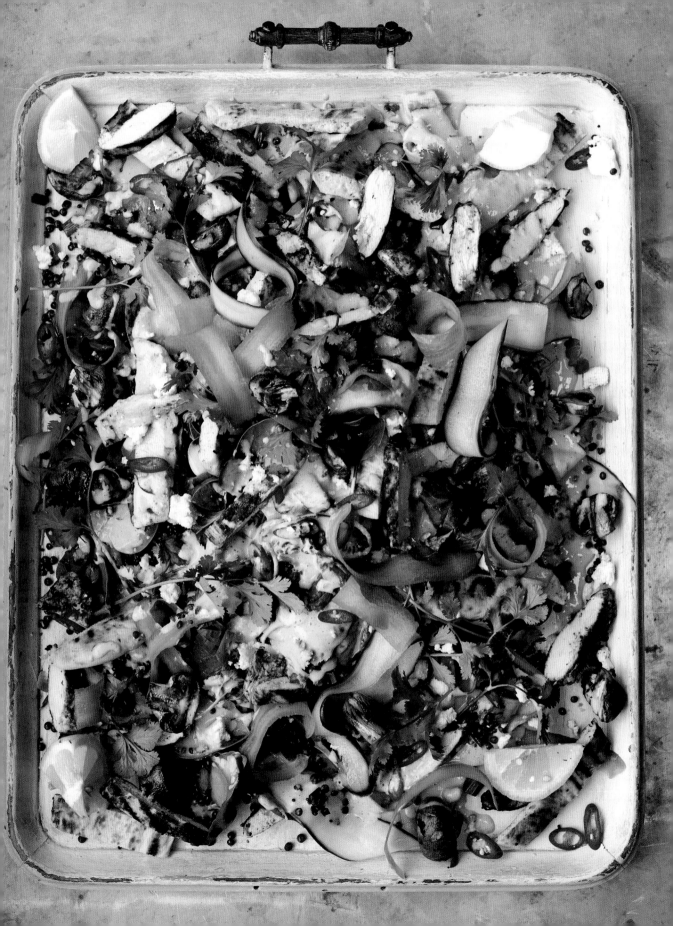

SPICY CAJUN CHICKEN
SMASHED SWEET POTATO & FRESH CORN SALSA

Ingredients out • *Kettle boiled* • *Griddle pan, high heat* • *Food processor (fine slicer)*
• *Large lidded pan, high heat* • *Large frying pan, medium-high heat*

Salsa
4 corn on the cob
1 small bunch of fresh coriander
1 fresh red chilli
4 spring onions
3 ripe tomatoes
2 limes
1 tbsp extra virgin olive oil

Smash
800g sweet potatoes
2 tbsp sweet chilli sauce

Chicken
4 x 120g skinless chicken breasts
1 tbsp Cajun seasoning
1 tbsp polenta
olive oil
2 rashers of smoked streaky bacon
175g okra
20g feta cheese

START COOKING

Put the corn on the griddle pan, turning when charred • Wash the sweet potatoes, remove any gnarly bits of skin with a speed-peeler, then finely slice in the processor • Put the sweet potatoes into the large pan, then just cover with boiling salted water and the lid • On a large sheet of greaseproof paper, toss the chicken with salt, the Cajun seasoning and polenta • Fold over the paper, then bash and flatten the chicken to 1.5cm thick with a rolling pin

Put the chicken into the frying pan with 2 tablespoons of olive oil, turning after 3 or 4 minutes, until golden and cooked through • Drain the cooked sweet potatoes well, return to the pan and mash with the sweet chilli sauce, pop the lid on and leave on a very low heat • Slice the bacon and add to the frying pan • As soon as the bacon starts to crisp up, add the okra to the pan

Carefully hold the charred corn steady and run a knife down the sides to cut off the kernels, then put them into a bowl • Roughly chop the top leafy half of the coriander and add to the corn • Finely slice the chilli and trimmed spring onions, chop the tomatoes, and add to the bowl with a pinch of salt, the lime juice and extra virgin olive oil, then mix well • Serve the sweet potato smash on a board or platter with the chicken and okra, crumble over the feta, and serve with the fresh salsa on the side

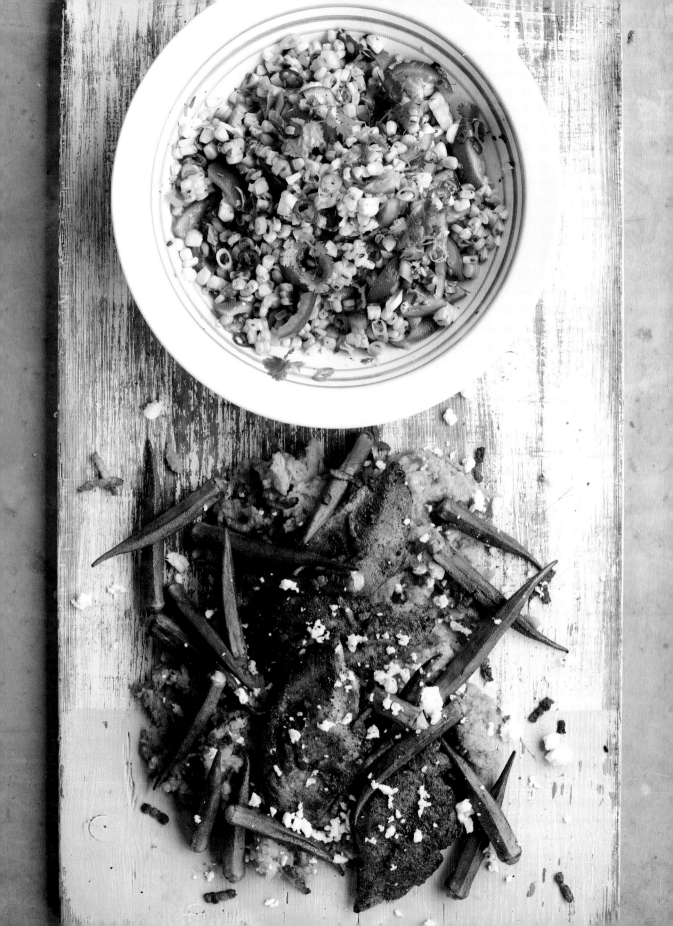

INCREDIBLY DELICIOUS
CHICKEN SALAD

SERVES 4 | 557 CALORIES

*Ingredients out • Kettle boiled • Medium lidded pan, high heat
• Frying pan, high heat • Griddle pan, high heat*

Salad

1 head of broccoli
4 x 120g skinless chicken breasts
1 heaped tsp ground coriander
olive oil
1 mug (300g) of bulgur wheat
2 preserved lemons
1 bunch of radishes
2 spring onions
½ a bunch of fresh mint
2 tbsp extra virgin olive oil
3 tbsp red wine vinegar
2 tbsp sunflower seeds
1 punnet of cress

To serve

4 tbsp fat-free natural yoghurt
2 tsp harissa
1 lemon

START COOKING

Fill the medium pan with boiling salted water • Trim the end off the broccoli stalk, then cut up the broccoli head and add to the pan, cover and boil for 4 minutes • On a large sheet of greaseproof paper, toss the chicken with salt, pepper and the ground coriander, then fold the paper over and bash and flatten to 1.5cm thick with a rolling pin • Put into the frying pan with 2 tablespoons of olive oil, turning after 3 or 4 minutes, until golden and cooked through

With tongs, remove and drain the broccoli (leaving the pan of water on the heat), then place on the griddle until nicely charred • Add 1 mug of bulgur wheat and the preserved lemons to the broccoli water and cover, stirring occasionally • Halve or crush the radishes, trim and finely slice the spring onions and the top leafy half of the mint, then toss it all in a bowl with the extra virgin olive oil and vinegar, and season to taste

Drain the bulgur wheat and tip into a large serving bowl, then mash and mix in the preserved lemons and arrange the broccoli on top • Toss the sunflower seeds in the chicken pan, then slice the chicken and add to the salad, scattering over the seeds and snipping over the cress • Serve dolloped with the yoghurt and drizzles of harissa, with lemon wedges on the side

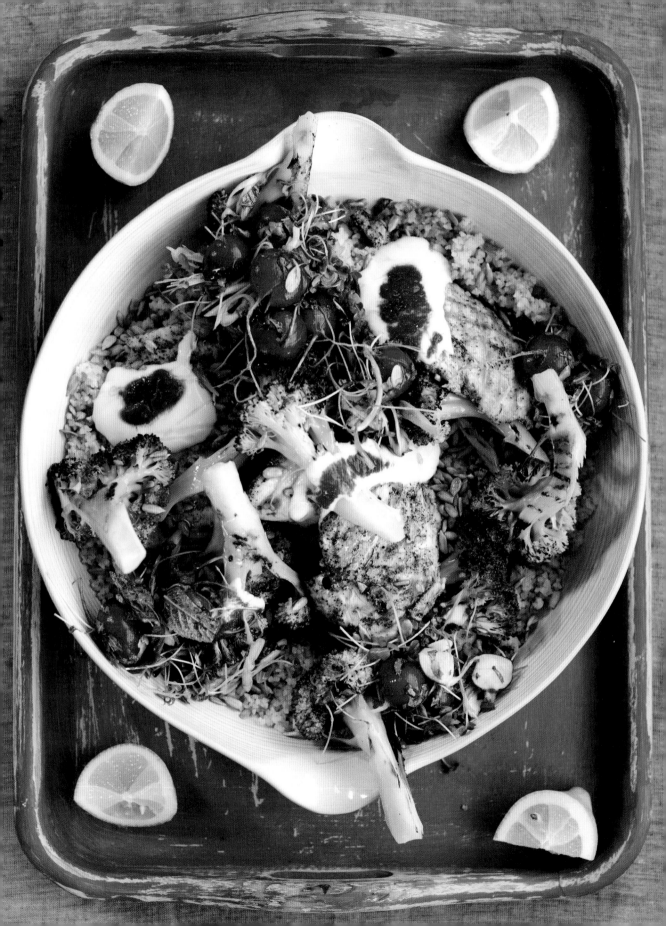

SIZZLING CHICKEN FAJITAS
GRILLED PEPPERS, SALSA, RICE & BEANS

Ingredients out • Kettle boiled • Liquidizer • Griddle pan, high heat
• Medium frying pan, medium-high heat • Large pan, medium heat

Salsa

1 dried smoked chipotle
   or ancho chilli
2 spring onions
1 ripe large tomato
½ a bunch of fresh coriander
1 fresh red chilli
2 limes
2 tsp balsamic vinegar
1 tbsp low-salt soy sauce

Fajitas

2 mixed-colour peppers
1 red onion
2 x 200g skinless chicken breasts
1 heaped tsp sweet smoked
   paprika, plus extra to serve
olive oil

Rice & beans

1 x 400g tin of mixed beans
½ tsp cumin seeds
1 fresh red chilli
1 x 250g pack of cooked brown rice
1 lemon

To serve

4 wholemeal flour tortillas
4 tbsp fat-free natural yoghurt
20g feta cheese

START COOKING

Tear the dried chilli into the liquidizer and just cover with boiling water to rehydrate • Trim and add the spring onions with the tomato, coriander stalks, fresh chilli, juice of 1 lime, the balsamic and soy sauce, pop the lid on and leave to sit • Remove the stalks and seeds from the peppers, then tear up and place on the griddle pan • Peel, quarter and add the red onion, season with salt and pepper, then let it char nicely all over

On a large sheet of greaseproof paper, toss the chicken with salt, pepper and the paprika • Fold over the paper, then bash and flatten the chicken to 1.5cm thick with a rolling pin • Put into the frying pan with 1 tablespoon of oil, turning after 3 or 4 minutes, until golden and cooked through • Drain and rinse the beans, then put into the large pan with 1 tablespoon of oil, the cumin seeds and the whole fresh chilli • Toss regularly for a couple of minutes until the beans are crispy-skinned

Whiz the contents of the liquidizer until smooth, then pour into a little serving bowl • Stir the rice and the juice of 1 lemon into the beans to warm through • Transfer the charred veg to a board, then merely warm the tortillas on the griddle pan • Slice the chicken and serve with the charred veg, rice and beans, tortillas and lime wedges • Dollop yoghurt over the veg, then sprinkle everything with crumbled feta and the coriander leaves

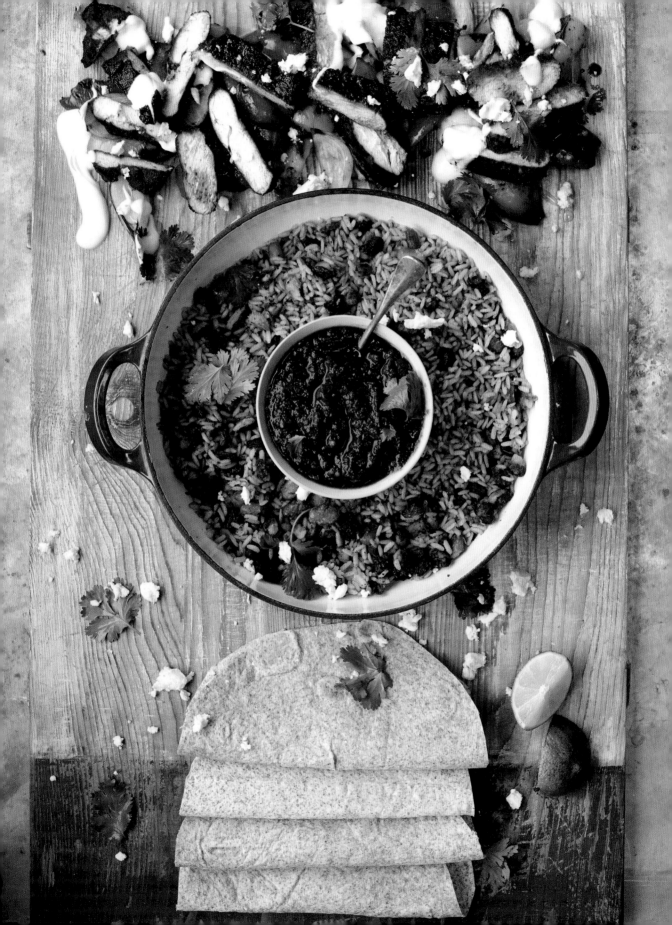

STICKY KICKING CHICKEN
WATERMELON RADISH SALAD & CRUNCHY NOODLES

SERVES 4 | 694 CALORIES

Ingredients out • Kettle boiled • Large frying pan, high heat
• Medium frying pan, medium heat • Liquidizer

Salad
200g thin rice noodles
sesame oil
800g watermelon
2 little gem lettuces
1 handful of radishes
½ a bunch of fresh mint
½ a bunch of fresh coriander

Chicken
8 skinless, boneless chicken thighs
1 tbsp Chinese five-spice
olive oil
2 tbsp sweet chilli sauce
2 tbsp sesame seeds

Dressing
2 tbsp low-salt soy sauce
1 tbsp fish sauce
½–1 fresh red chilli
½ a thumb-sized piece of ginger
2 spring onions
2 limes
1 small clove of garlic

START COOKING

In a bowl, fully submerge the noodles in boiling water • On a large sheet of greaseproof paper, toss the chicken with salt, pepper and the five-spice • Fold over the paper, then bash and flatten the chicken to 1.5cm thick with a rolling pin • Put into the large frying pan with 1 tablespoon of olive oil, turning after 3 or 4 minutes, until nicely charred and cooked through • Drain the noodles and toss with 1 tablespoon of sesame oil on a big serving platter • Put ¼ of the noodles into the medium frying pan, tossing regularly until nice and crunchy

Remove the watermelon skin, cut the flesh into erratic chunks and add to the platter • Trim the lettuces and cut into small wedges, halve the radishes, finely slice the top leafy half of the mint and most of the top leafy half of the coriander, and scatter over the platter • Put the coriander stalks into the liquidizer with the soy and fish sauces, chilli, peeled ginger, trimmed spring onions, a splash of water, 1 tablespoon of sesame oil and the lime juice • Squash in the unpeeled garlic through a garlic crusher, then whiz until smooth

Drain away any excess fat from the chicken pan, put back on the heat, drizzle with the sweet chilli sauce and toss with the sesame seeds • Pour the dressing over the salad and toss gently with clean fingers until well coated, then break over the crispy noodles • Transfer the chicken to a board and serve with an extra sprinkling of coriander leaves

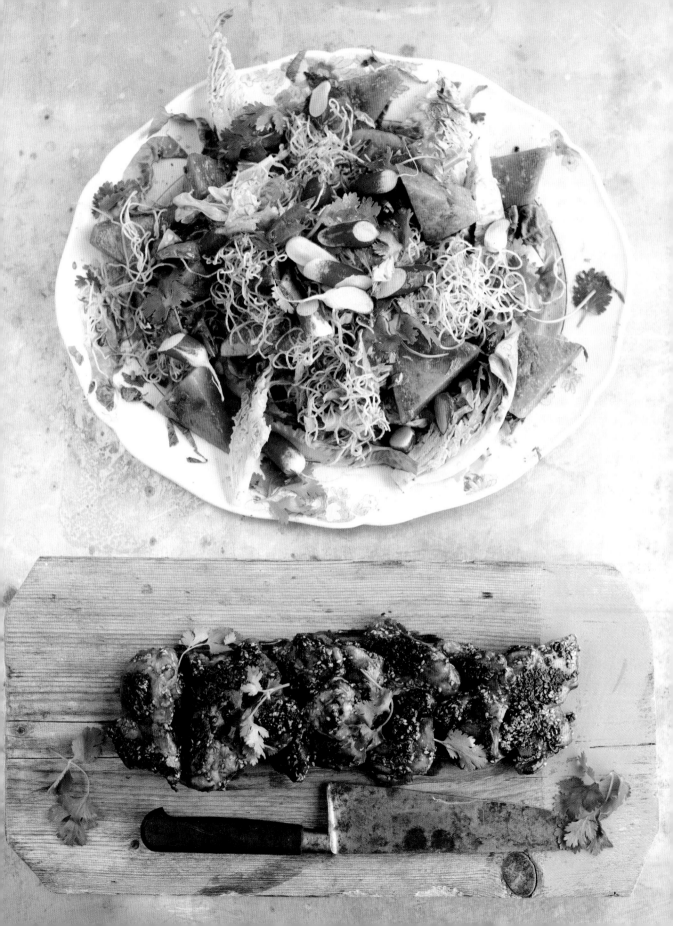

MEXICAN CHICKEN
WICKED MOLE SAUCE, RICE & VEG

SERVES 4 | 625 CALORIES

Ingredients out • Kettle boiled • Lidded casserole pan, medium heat • Medium lidded pan, medium heat • Liquidizer • Medium frying pan, low heat

Chicken, rice & veg

2 carrots

2 spring onions

2 chicken stock cubes

1 red pepper

2 rashers of smoked streaky bacon

a couple of sprigs of fresh thyme

1 mug (300g) of 10-minute
   wholegrain or basmati rice

4 x 120g skinless chicken breasts

175g okra

100g frozen peas

Mole sauce

3 spring onions

2 cloves of garlic

½ a fresh red chilli

1 dried smoked chipotle
   or ancho chilli

1 pinch of cumin seeds

1 heaped tbsp smooth peanut
   butter

30g dark chocolate
   (70% cocoa solids)

1 heaped tsp cocoa powder

a 2.5cm piece of banana

1 lemon

START COOKING

Finely slice the carrots and trimmed spring onions, then put into the casserole pan with 500ml of boiling water and crumble in the stock cubes • Deseed the pepper, cut into 8, then add to the stock with the bacon and thyme sprigs and put the lid on • Put 1 mug of rice and 2 mugs of boiling water into the medium pan with a pinch of salt and cover with a lid, stirring occasionally

Trim and add the spring onions, peeled garlic and chillies to the liquidizer with the cumin seeds, peanut butter, a couple of splashes of boiling water, salt and pepper, then blitz until fine • Put into the frying pan, boil, then simmer • Add the chicken, okra and peas to the casserole pan until the chicken is cooked through, replace the lid

Scrape the mixture from the frying pan back into the liquidizer and add the chocolate, cocoa, peeled banana and lemon juice, then whiz until silky smooth and season until it's incredible • Fluff up the rice, finely slice the chicken and serve with the mole sauce, veg and broth

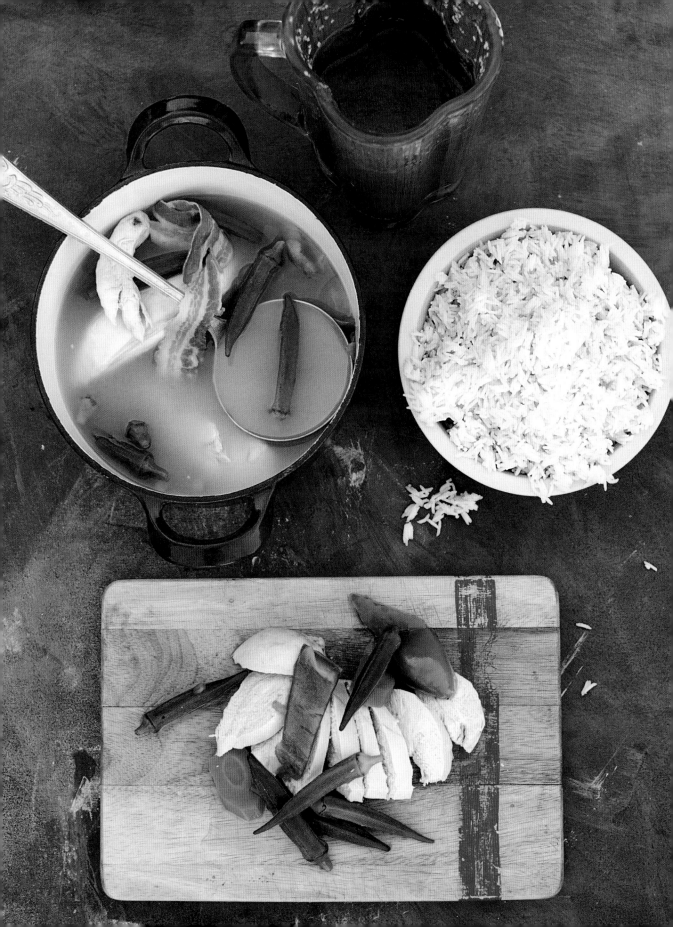

GORGEOUS GREEK CHICKEN
HERBY VEGETABLE COUSCOUS & TZATZIKI

SERVES 4 | 683 CALORIES

Ingredients out • Kettle boiled • Large frying pan, medium-high heat
• Food processor (bowl blade)

Couscous

1 mug (300g) of couscous
2 mixed-colour peppers
1 fresh red chilli
4 spring onions
½ a bunch of fresh dill
200g podded raw or frozen peas
1 small handful of black olives
  (stone in)
2 tbsp extra virgin olive oil
40g feta cheese

Chicken

2 x 200g skinless chicken breasts
1 heaped tsp dried oregano
1 tsp ground allspice
1 lemon
olive oil

Tzatziki

½ a cucumber
250g fat-free natural yoghurt
½ a lemon
½ a bunch of fresh mint

START COOKING

Put 1 mug of couscous and 2 mugs of boiling water into a bowl with a pinch of salt and cover • On a large sheet of greaseproof paper, toss the chicken with salt, pepper, the oregano, allspice and finely grated lemon zest • Fold over the paper, then bash and flatten the chicken to 1.5cm thick with a rolling pin • Put into the frying pan with 2 tablespoons of olive oil, turning after 3 or 4 minutes, until golden and cooked through

Using a box grater, coarsely grate the cucumber • Sprinkle it with a good pinch of salt, then squeeze and scrunch with clean hands to get rid of the excess salty water • Pop in a bowl with the yoghurt, juice of ½ a lemon and a pinch of pepper, finely chop and add the top leafy half of the mint, then mix together • Remove the stalk and seeds from the peppers and chilli, then pulse in the processor with the trimmed spring onions and the dill until finely chopped • Scatter over a large tray or platter

Add the peas to the veg (if using frozen peas, blanch them in boiling water for a couple of minutes first), destone and tear over the olives, then squeeze over the juice of the zested lemon and add the extra virgin olive oil • Fluff up and scatter over the couscous, toss well and season to taste • Move the cooked chicken to a board, slice it up, then lay it around the couscous • Crumble over the feta and serve with the tzatziki

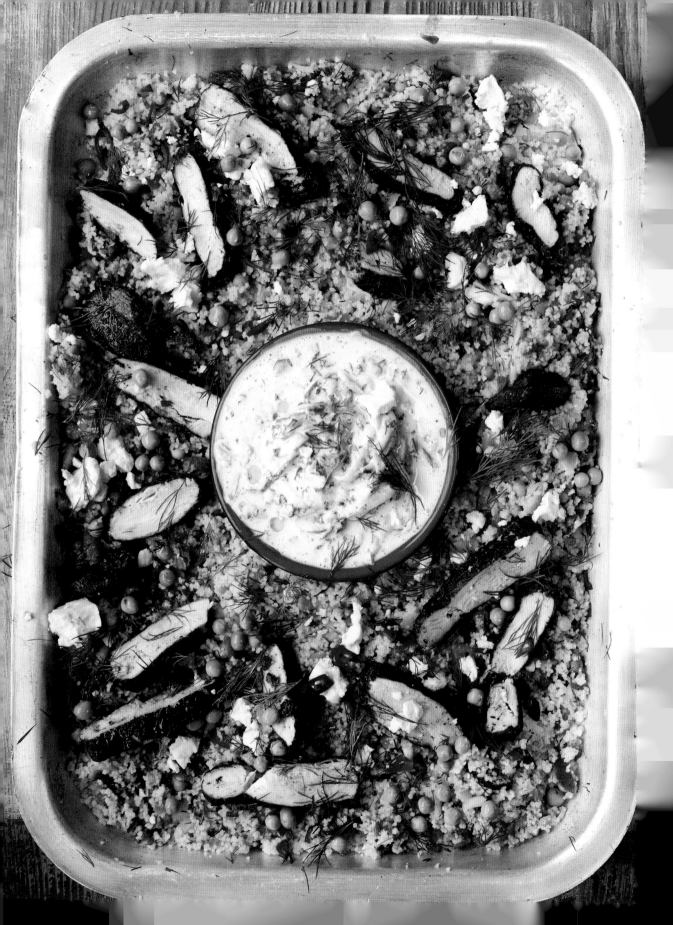

ROSEMARY CHICKEN
GRILLED POLENTA & PORCINI TOMATO SAUCE

Ingredients out • Kettle boiled • Liquidizer • Medium lidded pan, medium heat • Griddle pan, high heat • Frying pan, medium heat

Sauce
1 big pinch of dried porcini
   mushrooms
400g ripe vine tomatoes
1 heaped tbsp tomato purée
½ a fresh red chilli
1 bunch of fresh basil
2 cloves of garlic

Chicken & polenta
500g ready-made polenta
olive oil
1 bunch of asparagus (300g)
2 x 200g skinless chicken breasts
a few sprigs of fresh rosemary
½ tbsp fennel seeds
20g Parmesan cheese
4 rashers of smoked pancetta
150g oyster mushrooms
200g baby spinach
balsamic vinegar

START COOKING

Put the porcini in the liquidizer with 150ml of boiling water, the tomatoes, tomato purée, chilli and basil, squash in the unpeeled garlic through a garlic crusher and blitz until smooth • Pour the tomato sauce into the medium pan and boil for 8 minutes, stirring occasionally • Cut the polenta into 8 slices, rub with salt, pepper and 1 teaspoon of oil and place on the griddle pan, flipping over when charred and placing the trimmed asparagus on top of the polenta to steam

On a large sheet of greaseproof paper, toss the chicken with salt, pepper, the rosemary leaves, fennel seeds, and finely grated Parmesan • Fold the paper over, then bash and flatten the chicken to 1.5cm thick with a rolling pin • Put into the frying pan with 1 tablespoon of oil, turning after 3 or 4 minutes, until golden and cooked through • Toss the pancetta and mushrooms into the pan when you turn the chicken

Season the sauce to taste, pour on to a nice serving platter and top with the polenta slices and asparagus • Transfer the chicken, pancetta and mushrooms to a board while you quickly wilt the spinach in the frying pan • Season the spinach to taste and add to the platter • Slice the chicken and arrange on top with the pancetta and mushrooms, then drizzle everything with balsamic vinegar

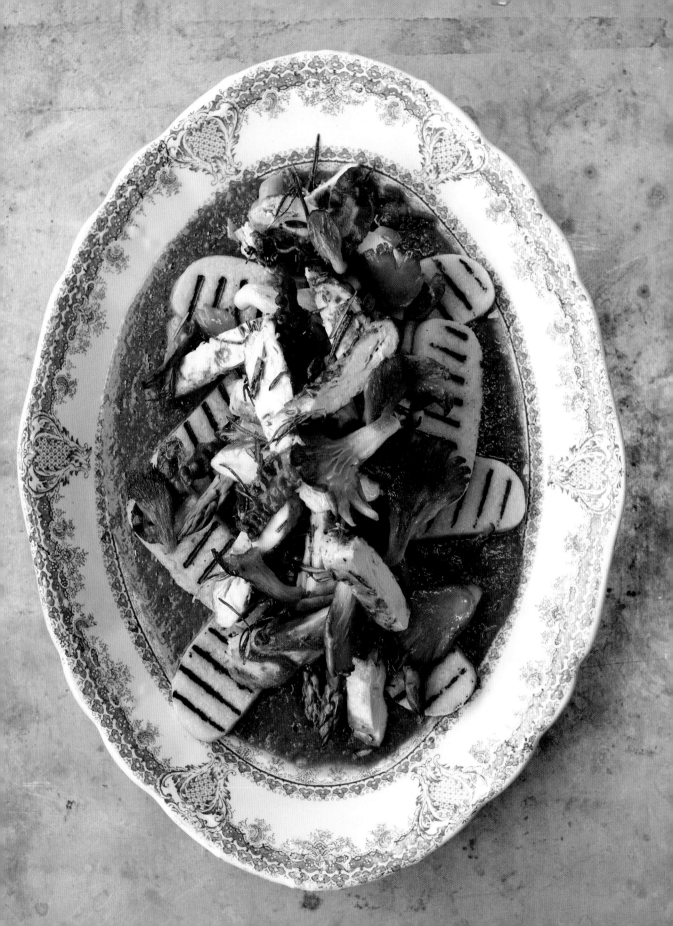

WARM CHICKEN LIVER SALAD
LITTLE WELSH 'RAREBITES'

SERVES 4 | 607 CALORIES

Ingredients out • Oven grill at full whack • Food processor (fine slicer) • Large frying pan, medium heat

'Rarebites'

1 ciabatta loaf
100g Cheddar cheese
4 tbsp fat-free natural yoghurt
2 tsp wholegrain mustard
1 tbsp Worcestershire sauce
Tabasco

Salad

1 small red onion
½ a cucumber
1 carrot
1 lemon
2 tbsp extra virgin olive oil
½ a bunch of fresh flat-leaf parsley
200g mixed salad leaves
50g alfalfa sprouts
balsamic vinegar
10g feta cheese

Livers

2 rashers of smoked streaky bacon
olive oil
400g chicken livers,
    cleaned and trimmed
2 sprigs of fresh rosemary
1 tsp marmalade
125ml Marsala
2 tbsp fat-free natural yoghurt

START COOKING

Cut the ciabatta into 8 thick slices • Put them on a large baking tray and lightly toast under the grill on both sides • Finely grate the Cheddar into a bowl and mix with the yoghurt, mustard, Worcestershire sauce and a few drips of Tabasco • Spoon over the toasts and return to the grill on the middle shelf, removing when golden and crisp (keep an eye on them)

Peel the onion, then finely slice in the processor with the cucumber and carrot • Tip into a bowl, squeeze over the lemon juice, add the extra virgin olive oil and season with salt and pepper, then tear over the top leafy half of the parsley • Turn the heat under the frying pan up to high, then slice the bacon and put into the pan with 1 tablespoon of olive oil, the chicken livers and rosemary leaves • Toss regularly for 3 minutes, season with salt and pepper, add the marmalade and Marsala, carefully light it with a match (if you want), let the flames subside, and cook until sticky, then remove from the heat and marble in the yoghurt

Toss the salad leaves and alfalfa sprouts with the dressed sliced veg, drizzle with balsamic and spread over a large platter • Crumble over the feta and arrange the 'rarebites' around the edge • Serve with the pan of chicken livers on the side

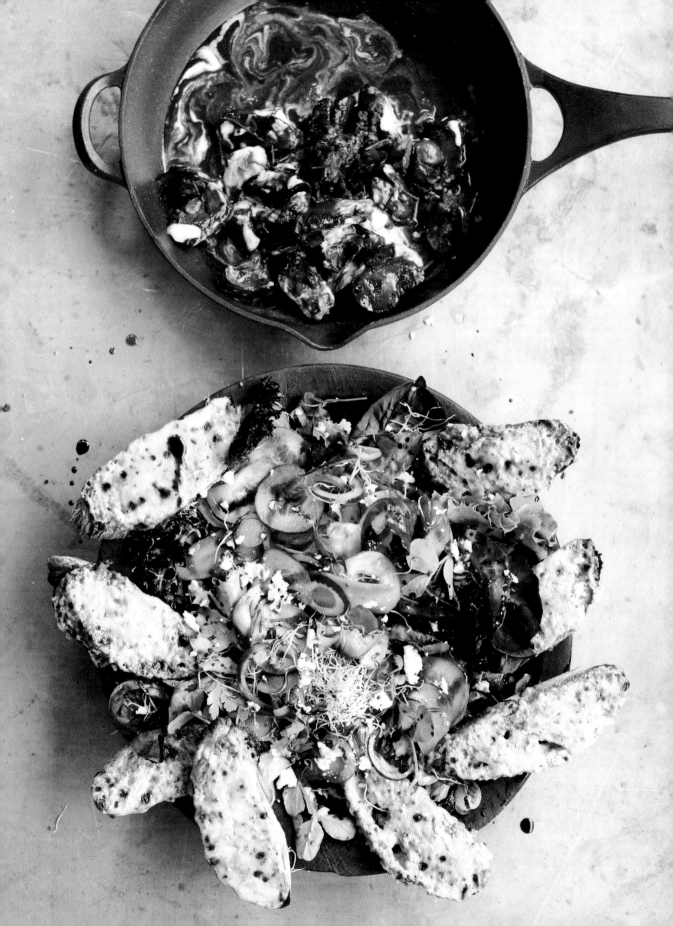

THAI CHICKEN LAKSA
MILDLY SPICED NOODLE SQUASH BROTH

SERVES 4 | 656 CALORIES

Ingredients out ⋅ Kettle boiled ⋅ Griddle pan, high heat
⋅ Large lidded pan, high heat ⋅ Food processor (coarse grater & bowl blade)

Chicken

4 skinless, boneless chicken thighs
1 heaped tsp Chinese five-spice
1 tbsp runny honey
1 tbsp sesame seeds
1 fresh red chilli

Laksa

1 chicken or vegetable stock cube
1 butternut squash (neck end only)
2 cloves of garlic
1 thumb-sized piece of ginger
1 fresh red chilli
1 tsp turmeric
½ a bunch of spring onions
1 heaped tsp peanut butter
4 dried kaffir lime leaves
½ a bunch of fresh coriander
1 tbsp sesame oil
1 tbsp low-salt soy sauce
1 tbsp fish sauce
300g medium rice noodles
2 bunches of asparagus (600g)
1 x 400g tin of light coconut milk
3 limes

START COOKING

On a large sheet of greaseproof paper, toss the chicken with salt, pepper and the five-spice ⋅ Fold over the paper, then bash and flatten the chicken to 1.5cm thick with a rolling pin ⋅ Place on the hot griddle pan, turning after 3 or 4 minutes, until nicely charred and cooked through ⋅ Pour about 800ml of boiling water into the large pan and crumble in the stock cube

Trim the stalk off the squash, roughly chop the neck end (don't peel, and keep the seed end for another day), then grate and tip into the boiling stock ⋅ Swap to the bowl blade in the processor and add the peeled garlic and ginger, the chilli, turmeric, trimmed spring onions, peanut butter, dried lime leaves, coriander stalks (reserving the leaves), sesame oil, soy and fish sauces ⋅ Blitz to a paste, then tip into the stock and add the noodles

Trim the asparagus and cut in half ⋅ Add to the pan, pour in the coconut milk, and as soon as it boils, taste, correct the seasoning with soy sauce and lime juice, then turn the heat off ⋅ Drizzle the honey over the charred chicken, squeeze over the juice of 1 lime, scatter with the sesame seeds and toss to coat ⋅ Serve with the laksa and lime wedges, sprinkling everything with the coriander leaves and slices of fresh chilli

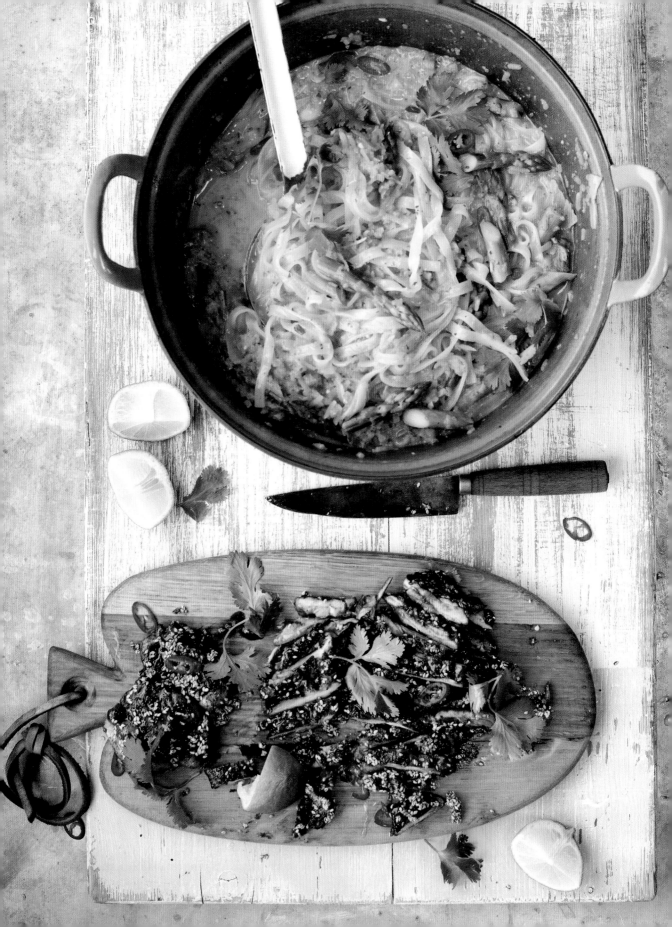

BLACKENED CHICKEN
SAN FRAN QUINOA SALAD

SERVES 4 | 617 CALORIES

Ingredients out • Kettle boiled • Medium lidded pan, medium-high heat • Food processor (bowl blade) • Large frying pan, high heat

Quinoa salad

1 mug (300g) of quinoa
1 fresh red or yellow chilli
100g baby spinach
4 spring onions
1 bunch of fresh coriander
1 bunch of fresh mint
1 ripe large mango
2 limes
2 tbsp extra virgin olive oil
1 ripe avocado
50g feta cheese
1 punnet of cress

Chicken

2 x 200g skinless chicken breasts
1 heaped tsp ground allspice
1 heaped tsp smoked paprika
olive oil
2 mixed-colour peppers

To serve

4 tbsp fat-free natural yoghurt

START COOKING

Put the quinoa into the pan and generously cover with boiling water and the lid • Put the chilli, spinach, trimmed spring onions and coriander (reserving a few leaves) into the processor, tear in the top leafy half of the mint, then blitz until finely chopped • On a large sheet of greaseproof paper, toss the chicken with salt, pepper, the allspice and paprika • Fold over the paper, then bash and flatten the chicken to 1.5cm thick with a rolling pin • Put into the frying pan with 1 tablespoon of olive oil, turning after 3 or 4 minutes, until blackened and cooked through

Deseed the peppers, cut each one into 8 strips and add to the frying pan, tossing regularly • Peel and cut the mango into chunks (check out: *www. jamieoliver.com/how-to* for a video of how to do this) • Drain the quinoa and rinse under the cold tap, then drain well again and tip on to a serving board or platter • Toss with the blitzed spinach mixture, squeeze over the lime juice, add the extra virgin olive oil, mix well and season to taste

Sprinkle the mango chunks and cooked peppers over the quinoa • Halve and destone the avocado, then use a teaspoon to scoop curls of it over the salad • Slice up the chicken, toss the slices in any juices and add to the salad • Crumble over the feta, scatter over the remaining coriander leaves and snip over the cress • Serve with dollops of yoghurt

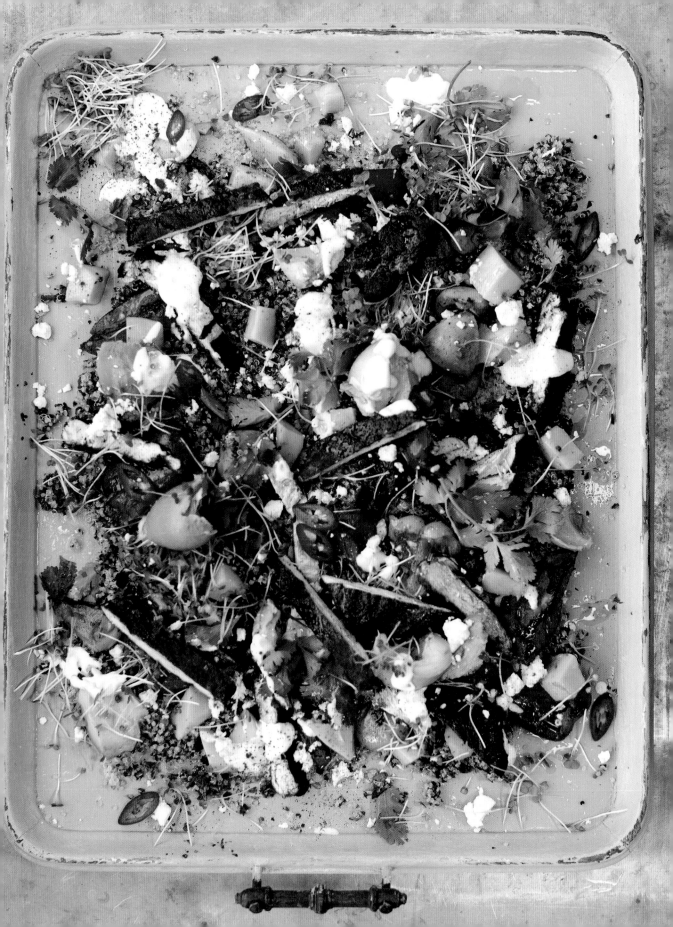

GOLDEN CHICKEN
BRAISED GREENS & POTATO GRATIN

SERVES 4 | 666 CALORIES

Ingredients out • *Kettle boiled* • *Oven grill on high* • *Food processor (fine slicer)*
• *Medium lidded pan, high heat* • *Large high-sided roasting tray, high heat*
• *Large frying pan, medium-high heat*

Gratin
800g potatoes
3 onions
olive oil
1 chicken stock cube
½ a bunch of fresh sage
100ml single cream
30g Parmesan cheese

Chicken
4 x 120g skinless chicken breasts
a few sprigs of fresh rosemary
2 rashers of smoked streaky bacon

Greens
200g baby leeks
200g baby spinach
200g frozen peas

START COOKING

Finely slice the potatoes in the processor, then tip into the medium pan and cover with boiling water and the lid • Peel the onions, finely slice in the processor, then tip into the roasting tray with 2 tablespoons of oil, crumble in the stock cube and season with salt and pepper • Tear in the sage leaves and stir regularly, adding a splash of water if they start to catch

On a large sheet of greaseproof paper, toss the chicken with salt, pepper and the rosemary leaves, then fold the paper over and bash and flatten the chicken to 1.5cm thick with a rolling pin • Put into the frying pan with 1 tablespoon of oil, turning after 3 or 4 minutes, until golden and cooked through • Drain the potatoes well in a colander, then tip into the onion pan, stir together and arrange in a flat layer • Pour over the cream, then finely grate over the Parmesan and pop under the grill on the top shelf

Halve the leeks lengthways, rinse under the tap, then finely slice • Put into the empty lidded pan on a high heat with 1 tablespoon of oil, stirring often • Finely slice the bacon and add to the chicken pan, tossing regularly • Stir the spinach and peas into the leeks and once the spinach has wilted and the peas are tender, pile on a board or platter with the chicken and bacon on top • Serve with the gratin

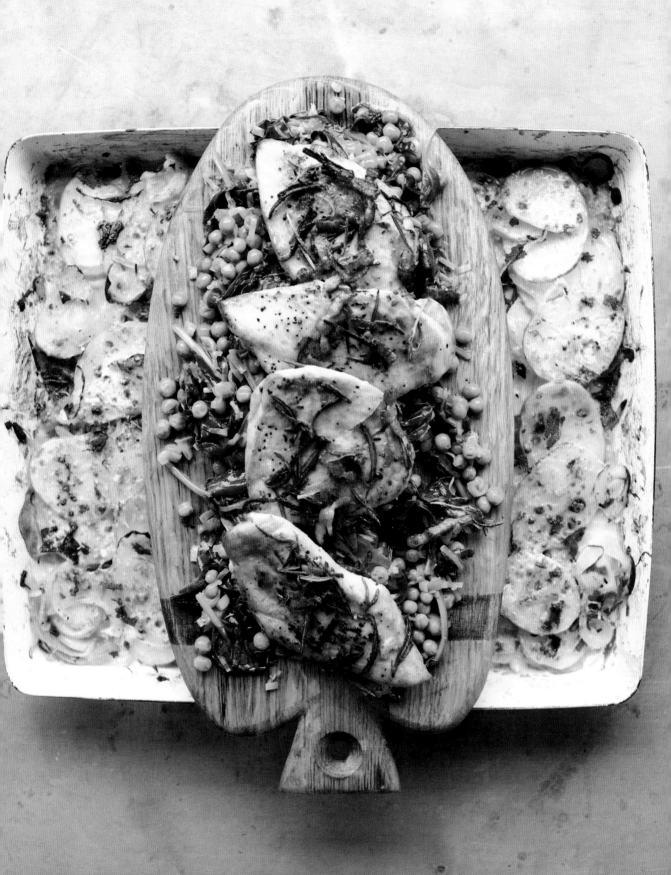

CRISPY POLENTA CHICKEN
CAESAR SALAD

SERVES 4 | 476 CALORIES

Ingredients out • *Large frying pan, medium heat*
• *Griddle pan, high heat* • *Liquidizer*

Chicken

2 x 200g skinless chicken breasts
½ tsp sweet smoked paprika
2 heaped tbsp polenta
olive oil

Salad

1 ciabatta loaf
1 clove of garlic
2 red chicory
4 slices of smoked pancetta
2 romaine lettuces
10 ripe cherry tomatoes
2 large jarred red peppers
balsamic vinegar
1 punnet of cress

Dressing

1 clove of garlic
2 lemons
40g Parmesan cheese,
  plus extra to serve
4 anchovy fillets
4 heaped tbsp fat-free
  natural yoghurt
1 splash of Worcestershire sauce
1 tbsp red wine vinegar
1 tsp English mustard
½ a bunch of fresh basil

START COOKING

On a large sheet of greaseproof paper, toss the chicken with salt, pepper, the paprika and polenta • Fold over the paper, then bash and flatten the chicken to roughly 1.5cm thick with a rolling pin • Put into the frying pan with 1 tablespoon of oil, turning after 3 or 4 minutes, until golden and cooked through • Cut 4 thick slices of ciabatta, place on the griddle pan, and remove when nicely charred on both sides

Squash the unpeeled garlic through a garlic crusher into the liquidizer • Squeeze in the lemon juice, crumble in the Parmesan and add the rest of the dressing ingredients • Blitz until smooth, then season to taste • Rub the toasts with a halved garlic clove and cut into soldiers • Quarter the chicory and add to the griddle pan with the pancetta to char for a couple of minutes

Roughly slice the lettuces and arrange over a large serving board or platter • Scatter over the ciabatta soldiers, halve the tomatoes and slice the peppers, then add to the board • Toss the chicory in a splash of balsamic and arrange on top • Slice the chicken, lay it around the salad, drizzle with the dressing, crumble over the crispy pancetta and snip over the cress • Use a speed-peeler to shave over a little extra Parmesan, if you like

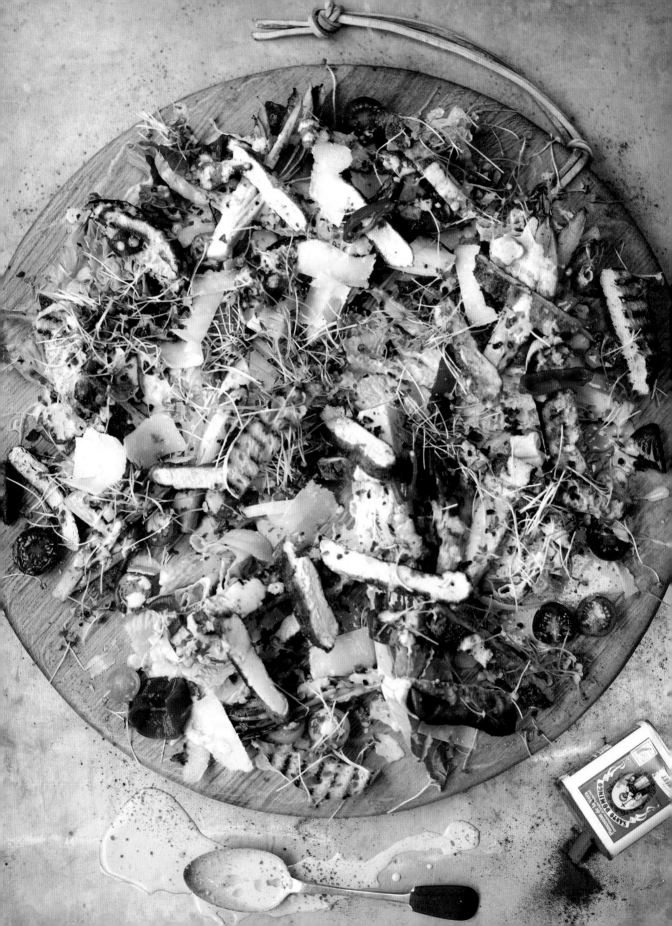

SPICED CHICKEN
BACON, ASPARAGUS & SPINACH LENTILS

Lentils

1 onion
1 carrot
2 sprigs of fresh rosemary
olive oil
2 x 400g tins of Puy lentils
1 ripe tomato
200g baby spinach
1 tsp red wine vinegar
4 heaped tbsp fat-free natural
   yoghurt

Chicken

4 x 120g skinless chicken breasts
½ tsp cayenne pepper
4 cloves of garlic
1 handful of fresh thyme,
   rosemary and/or bay
4 rashers of smoked pancetta
1 bunch of asparagus (300g)

To serve

crusty bread

Ingredients out • Food processor (bowl blade) • Oven at 180°C/350°F/gas 4 • Large lidded pan, medium heat • Large frying pan, medium heat

START COOKING

Peel and halve the onion and carrot, then blitz in the processor with the rosemary leaves until fine • Put into the large pan with 1 tablespoon of oil, tossing regularly • On a large sheet of greaseproof paper, toss the chicken with salt, pepper and the cayenne, then fold the paper over and bash and flatten to 1.5cm thick with a rolling pin • Put into the frying pan with 1 tablespoon of oil, the unpeeled whole garlic cloves and a handful of fresh herbs, turning after 3 or 4 minutes, until golden and cooked through

Stir the tinned lentils (and their juices) into the veg pan with the roughly chopped tomato and put the lid on • Pop the bread into the oven to warm through • Roughly chop the spinach in the processor and add to the lentils with the red wine vinegar • When the lentils are boiling and the spinach wilted, season to taste • Add the pancetta and trimmed asparagus to the chicken pan and fry until golden and crispy

Tip the lentils on to a platter, then marble through most of the yoghurt • Remove the chicken to a board, cut in half at an angle, and serve on top of the lentils with the crispy pancetta, asparagus and garlic • Dollop over the remaining yoghurt, then serve with the crusty bread to mop up the juices

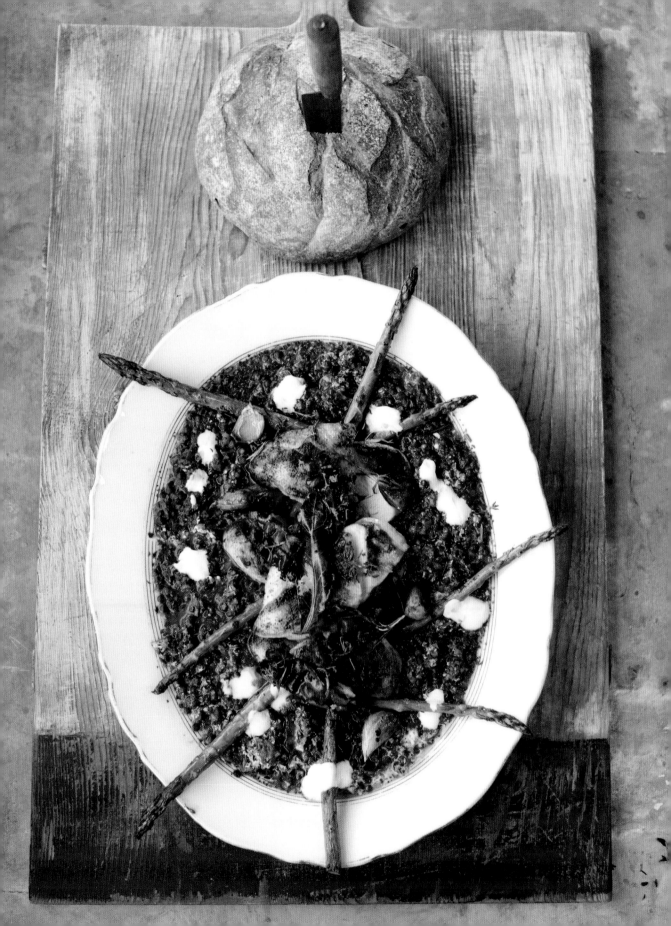

CRISPY DUCK
HOI SIN LETTUCE PARCELS

SERVES 4 | 738 CALORIES

Ingredients out • *Kettle boiled* • *Small lidded pan, medium heat*
• *Large frying pan, medium heat*

Parcels

4 nests of fine egg noodles
2 iceberg lettuces
1 tbsp sesame oil
4 tbsp hoi sin sauce
4 limes
1 clove of garlic
350g silken tofu
1 bunch of baby radishes
5 sprigs of fresh coriander
1 punnet of cress
sweet chilli sauce

Duck

2 x 200g duck breasts, skin on
1 heaped tsp Chinese five-spice
olive oil
1 fresh red chilli
2 spring onions
1 handful of cashew nuts
2 tbsp sesame seeds
1 tsp runny honey

START COOKING

Put the noodles into the small pan and cover with boiling water and the lid • Cut the duck into 1cm dice, toss with salt, pepper and the five-spice, then put into the frying pan with 1 tablespoon of olive oil and toss regularly • Cut the lettuces in half through the stalk, remove the stalk, then separate the leaves into cups and arrange on a large clean tray or platter

Drain the noodles and toss with the sesame oil, then divide them between the lettuce cups • Finely slice the chilli and trimmed spring onions • When the duck is nice and golden, pour away any excess fat, then stir in the chilli, spring onions, cashews and sesame seeds, and toss regularly

Put the hoi sin sauce into a bowl, squeeze in the juice from 3 limes, squash in the unpeeled garlic through a garlic crusher and mix together • Drizzle the duck with the honey, shake the pan to coat, then tip it evenly over the lettuce cups • Cut the tofu into rough 2cm chunks and sprinkle it in and around the lettuce cups • Scatter over the baby radishes and coriander leaves, then snip over the cress • Drizzle the hoi sin dressing over everything from a height and drizzle each piece of tofu with a little sweet chilli sauce • Serve with lime wedges

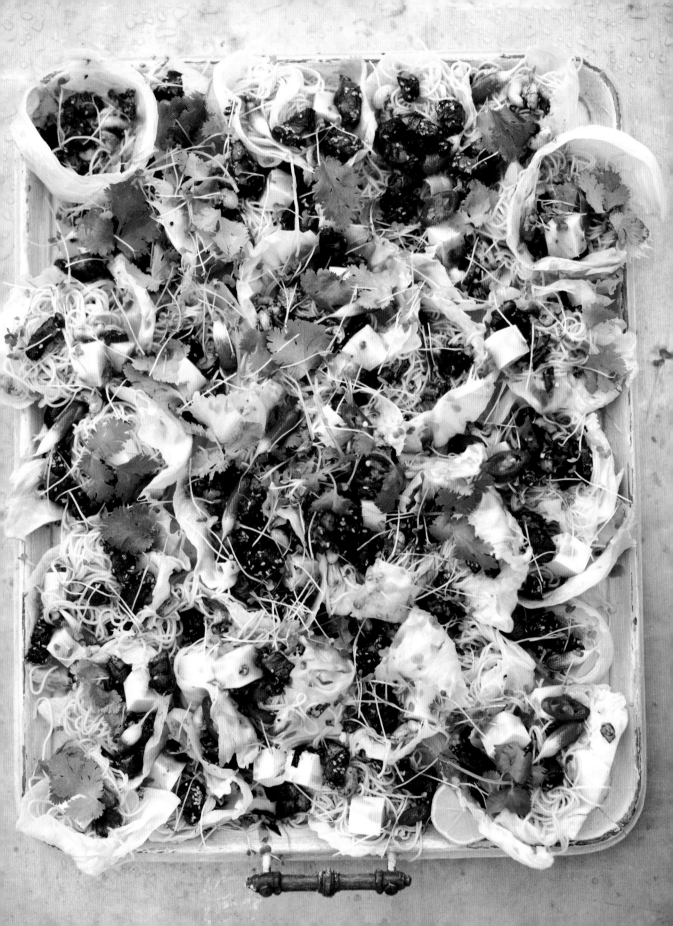

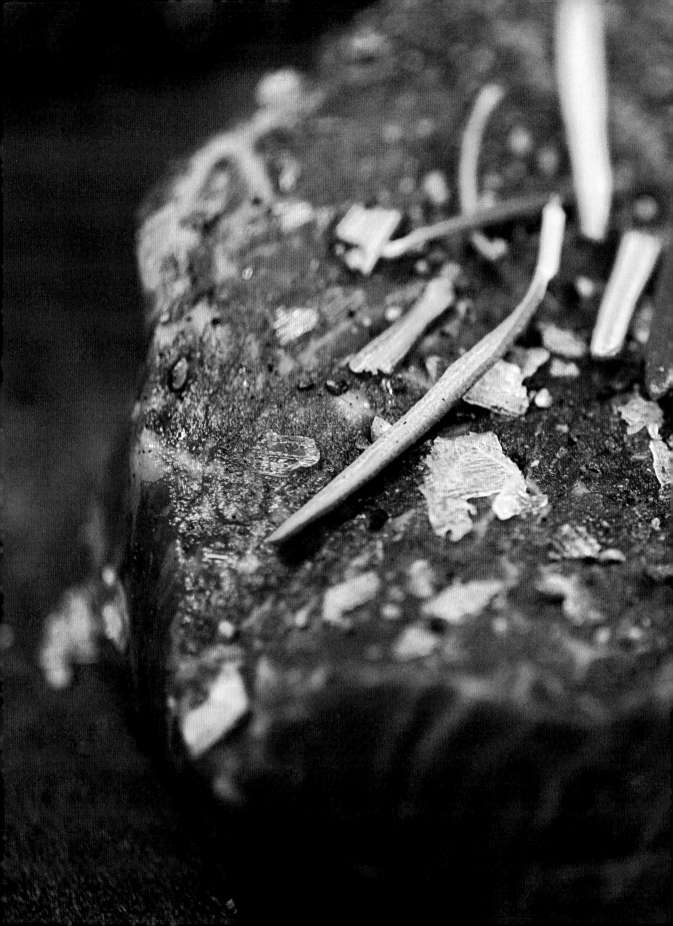

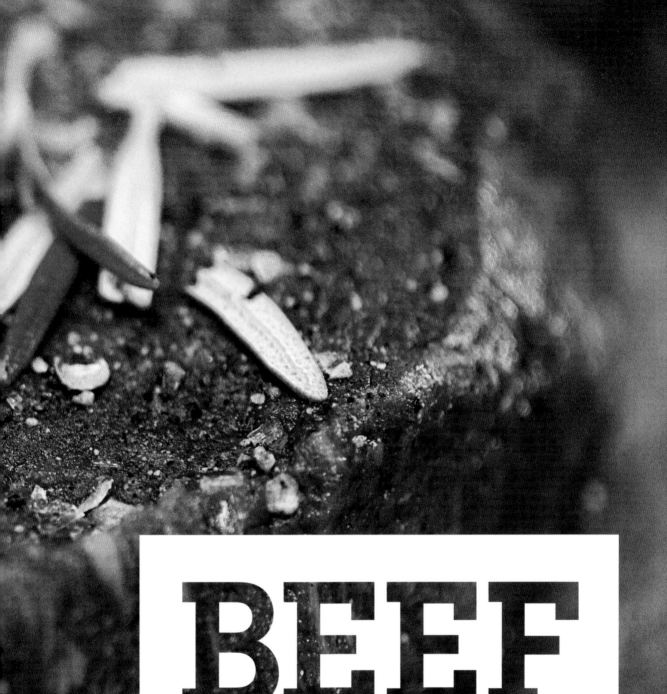

BEEF

CHILLI CON CARNE
MEATBALLS

SERVES 4 | 437 CALORIES

Ingredients out • Kettle boiled • Oven grill on high • Medium lidded pan, high heat • Large frying pan, high heat • Liquidizer • Medium frying pan, medium heat

Bulgur wheat

1 mug (300g) of bulgur wheat
1 preserved lemon
1 cinnamon stick

Meatballs

400g lean beef mince
1 heaped tsp garam masala
olive oil
3 jarred red peppers
4 spring onions
1 tsp smoked paprika
700g passata
1 bunch of fresh coriander
1 x 400g tin of red kidney beans
1 pinch of cumin seeds
4 tbsp fat-free natural yoghurt
1 lime

Grilled chillies

4 fresh chillies

START COOKING

Put 1 mug of bulgur wheat, 2 mugs of boiling water, the preserved lemon and the cinnamon stick into the medium pan and cover, stirring occasionally • With clean hands, scrunch the mince with salt, pepper and the garam masala • Divide the mixture into 4, then with wet hands quickly shape each piece into 4 balls, placing them into the frying pan as you roll them and adding 1 tablespoon of oil, toss regularly

Blitz the peppers, half the trimmed spring onions, the paprika, passata, half the coriander and a pinch of salt and pepper in the liquidizer until smooth, then pour into the medium frying pan (swirl a good splash of water around the liquidizer and pour into the pan) and turn the heat up to high • Prick the chillies and put under the grill to blacken all over, then remove

Rinse and drain the beans, then add to the meatballs with the cumin seeds • Use tongs to transfer the meatballs straight into the pan of sauce, leaving the beans behind • Finely slice the remaining trimmed spring onions • Stir the beans into the sauce • Remove the cinnamon stick, then mash the lemon into the bulgur wheat and serve with the meatball sauce, dollops of yoghurt, the charred chillies and wedges of lime, scattered with the remaining spring onions and coriander leaves

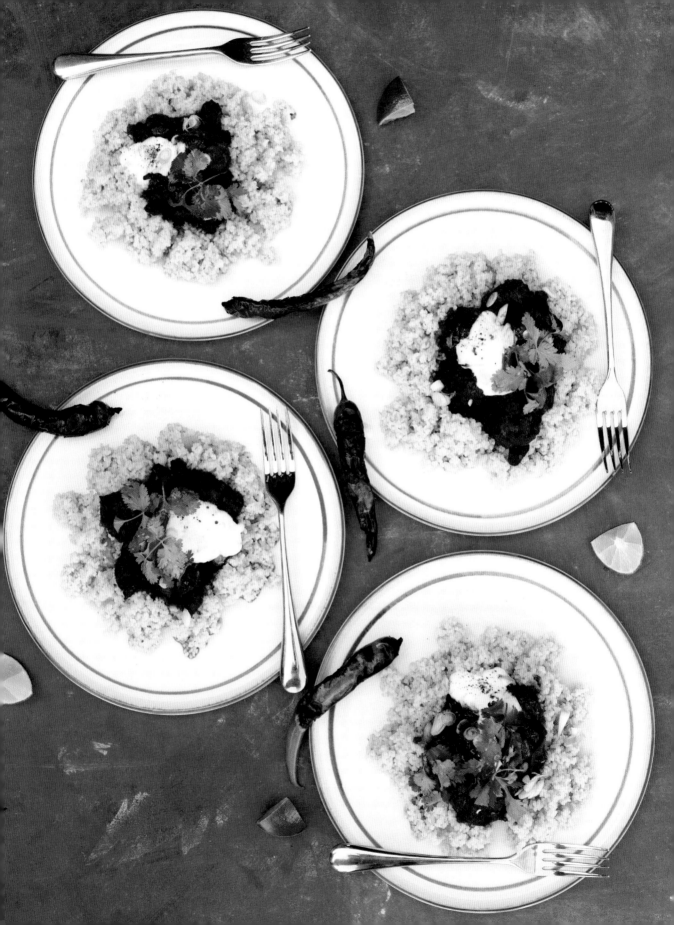

BRITISH BURGERS
SHRED SALAD, PICKLES & THINGS

SERVES 4 | 532 CALORIES

Ingredients out • Oven at 130°C/250°F/gas ½ • Large frying pan, medium heat • Food processor (coarse grater)

Burgers

500g lean beef mince
1 heaped tsp wholegrain mustard
1 swig of quality beer or ale
olive oil
4 wholewheat baps
2 tbsp fat-free natural yoghurt
Worcestershire sauce
1 ripe beef tomato
2–4 gherkins
tomato ketchup, to serve

Salad

2 carrots
¼ of a white cabbage
   (roughly 250g)
1 pear
1 small red onion
2 tbsp extra virgin olive oil
1 tbsp red wine vinegar
70g rocket

START COOKING

Put the mince into a bowl with salt, pepper, the mustard and the beer or ale, then with clean hands scrunch and mix together • Divide the mixture into 4 and with wet hands shape into patties about 2.5cm thick, then put into the pan with 1 tablespoon of olive oil, turning when crispy and golden, and pushing down on them with a fish slice so they're in good contact with the pan

Place the baps into the oven • Put the yoghurt into a small bowl, add a good splash of Worcestershire sauce, then stir and ripple it together • Slice the tomato and gherkins on a nice serving board

In the processor, grate the trimmed carrots, cabbage, pear (stalk removed) and peeled red onion • Put the extra virgin olive oil and vinegar into a serving bowl, tip in the grated veg, toss together and season to taste, then mix in the rocket • Get the baps out of the oven, cut them in half and dollop with ketchup • Top with a slice of tomato and the burgers, then let everyone build their own at the table

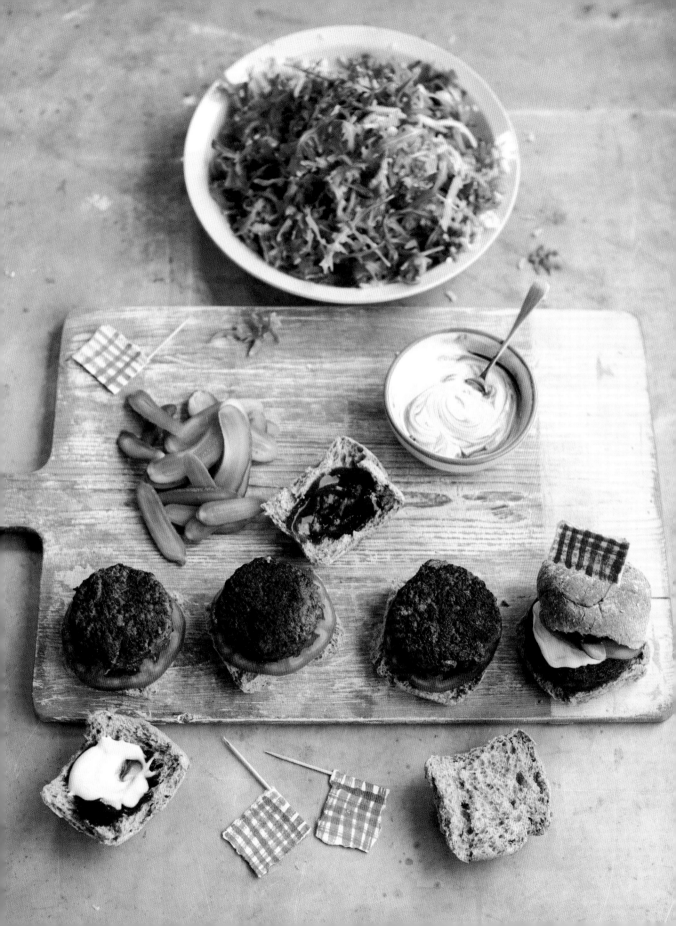

BEEF STROGANOFF
FLUFFY RICE, RED ONION & PARSLEY PICKLE

Ingredients out • Kettle boiled • Medium lidded pan, medium heat
• Food processor (fine slicer) • Large frying pan, high heat

Rice

1 mug (300g) of 10-minute
   wholegrain or basmati rice
½ a bunch of fresh thyme
200g baby spinach

Pickle

2 small red onions
1 handful of gherkins
1 bunch of fresh flat-leaf parsley

Stroganoff

300g mixed mushrooms
olive oil
3 cloves of garlic
2 x 200g sirloin steaks,
   fat removed
1 heaped tsp sweet paprika
1 lemon
1 swig of brandy
4 heaped tbsp fat-free natural
   yoghurt
1 swig of semi-skimmed milk

START COOKING

Put 1 mug of rice, 2 mugs of boiling water, the thyme leaves and a pinch of salt and pepper into the medium pan and put the lid on, stirring occasionally • Peel the onions, then finely slice them with the gherkins in the processor and tip into a bowl • Finely slice the parsley stalks and roughly chop the leaves, then toss into the bowl with a swig of gherkin vinegar and a pinch of salt, scrunching together well

Tear or slice the mushrooms into the frying pan with 2 tablespoons of oil, then squash in the unpeeled garlic through a garlic crusher and add two-thirds of the parsley pickle, stirring regularly • Slice the steaks about 1cm thick and toss with salt, pepper, the paprika and the finely grated lemon zest • Tip the mushrooms on to a plate, then add 2 tablespoons of oil and the steak to the pan in one layer, turning when golden

Add the spinach to the rice pan and replace the lid • Add the brandy to the steak, carefully light it with a match (if you want), let the flames subside, then return the mushrooms to the pan with the yoghurt and milk and bring to the boil • Transfer the wilted spinach to a nice serving platter, then fluff up and scatter the rice over the top • Spoon over the stroganoff, squeeze and drain the remaining pickle, then scatter over from a height

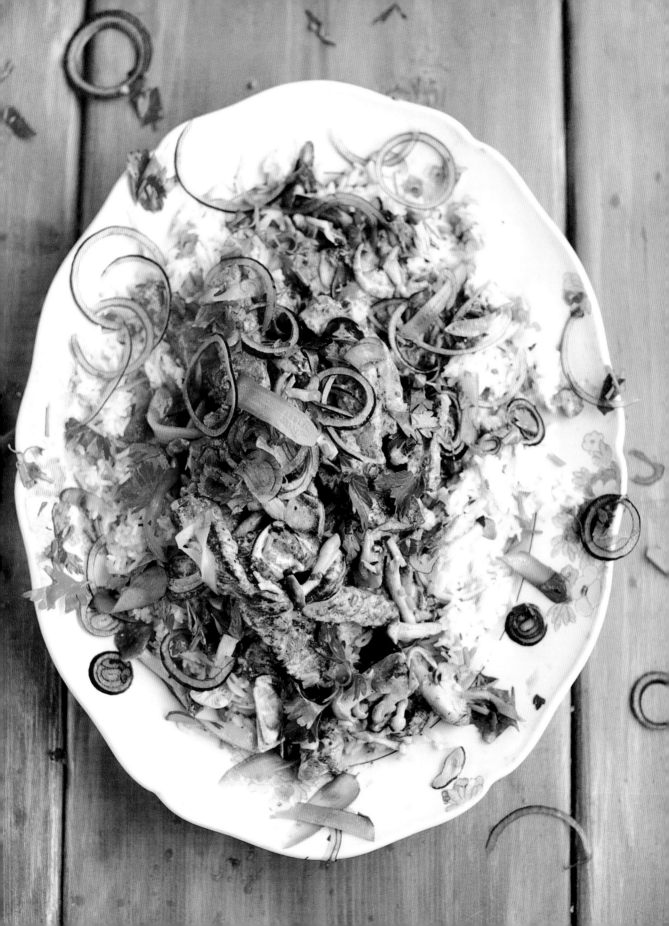

SIZZLING BEEF STEAK
HOI SIN PRAWN & NOODLE BOWLS

SERVES 4 | 653 CALORIES

Ingredients out • Kettle boiled • Wok, high heat • Large frying pan, high heat • Food processor (bowl blade) • Medium lidded pan, high heat

Bowls

2 tbsp shelled peanuts
2 tbsp sesame seeds
½–1 fresh red chilli
1 thumb-sized piece of ginger
2 spring onions
1 bunch of fresh coriander
4 nests of egg noodles
2 cloves of garlic
100g raw peeled tiger prawns
80g beansprouts
4 tbsp hoi sin sauce
2 tbsp low-salt soy sauce
2 limes
1 romaine lettuce
4 radishes
1 punnet of cress

Beef

2 x 200g sirloin steaks,
    fat removed
1 tbsp Chinese five-spice
2 tbsp sesame oil
250g oyster mushrooms

START COOKING

Toast the peanuts and sesame seeds in the dry wok, tossing often until golden, then tip into a small bowl and put aside, leaving the wok on the heat • Rub the steaks all over with salt, pepper and the five-spice, then put into the frying pan with half the sesame oil • Turn the steaks every minute until cooked to your liking, adding the mushrooms after a couple of minutes and removing the steaks to a board when done • Finely chop the chilli, peeled ginger, trimmed spring onions and half the coriander in the processor

Half-fill the pan with boiling salted water and add the noodles, then put the lid on • Put the remaining sesame oil into the wok, add the chopped veg and squash in the unpeeled garlic through a garlic crusher • Toss for a minute, add the prawns and beansprouts, toss for another minute, then add the hoi sin and soy sauces, the juice of 1 lime and the rest of the coriander leaves

Use tongs to drain and transfer the noodles straight into the wok and toss in, loosening with a splash of cooking water if needed • Season to taste and divide between 4 bowls • Trim the lettuce, break the leaves apart and poke a couple of leaves into each bowl with a halved radish • Snip over the cress and sprinkle with the toasted nuts and seeds • Cut the steaks into 1cm slices and serve with the crispy mushrooms and lime wedges

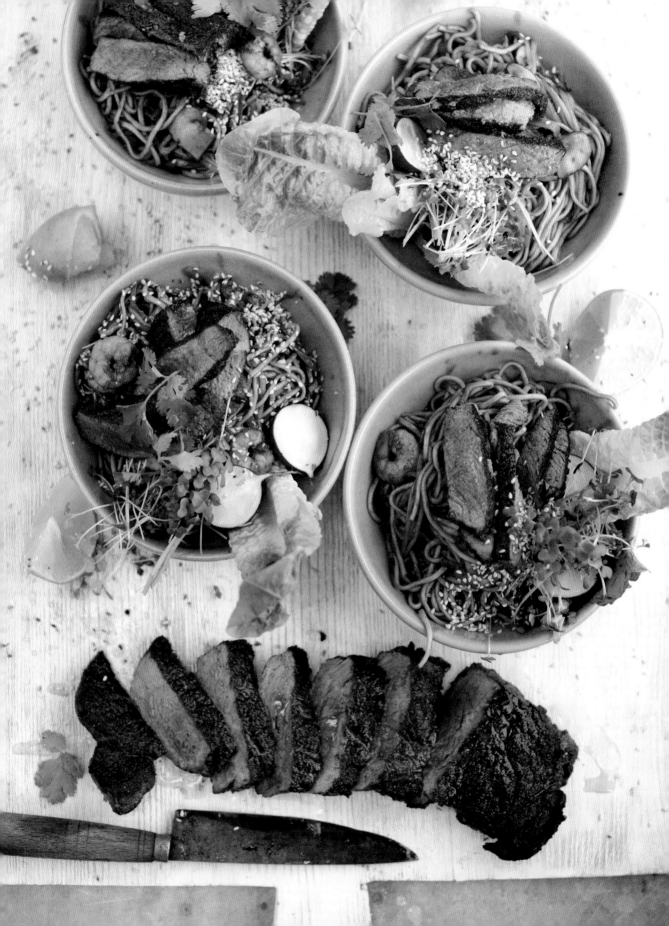

BEEF KOFTA CURRY
FLUFFY RICE, BEANS & PEAS

SERVES 4 | 706 CALORIES

Ingredients out • Kettle boiled • Large frying pan, high heat
• Medium lidded casserole pan, high heat • Liquidizer

Curry

1 x 250g pack of
    ready-to-eat Puy lentils
1 heaped tsp garam masala
400g lean beef mince
olive oil
3 ripe tomatoes
1 thumb-sized piece of ginger
2 spring onions
1 fresh red chilli
1 bunch of fresh coriander
1 tsp turmeric
1 tsp runny honey
2 heaped tsp Patak's rogan josh
    curry paste
½ x 400g tin of light coconut milk
4 tbsp fat-free natural yoghurt,
    to serve
1 lemon

Rice

1 mug (300g) of 10-minute
    wholegrain or basmati rice
5 cardamom pods
200g green or yellow beans
200g frozen peas
2 uncooked poppadoms

START COOKING

Put the lentils into a bowl with salt, pepper, the garam masala and mince, then mix and scrunch together with clean hands • Divide the mixture in half, then with wet hands quickly squeeze and mould each half into 6 fat fingers • Put them into the frying pan with 1 tablespoon of oil, turning when golden

Put 1 mug of rice, 2 mugs of boiling water and the cardamom pods into the casserole pan, then halve and add the beans and put the lid on • Squash the tomatoes into the liquidizer, add the peeled ginger, trimmed spring onions, half the chilli, the coriander stalks, turmeric, honey, curry paste and coconut milk, then blitz until combined • Pour into the kofta pan, bring to the boil, then simmer and season to taste

Take the lid off the rice, add the peas, mix it all up and give it just a few more minutes • Crack up the uncooked poppadoms and pop them in the microwave (800W) for a minute or two to puff up • Finely slice the remaining chilli and the coriander leaves and scatter them over the curry, dollop with yoghurt, then serve with lemon wedges, poppadoms and the rice, beans and peas

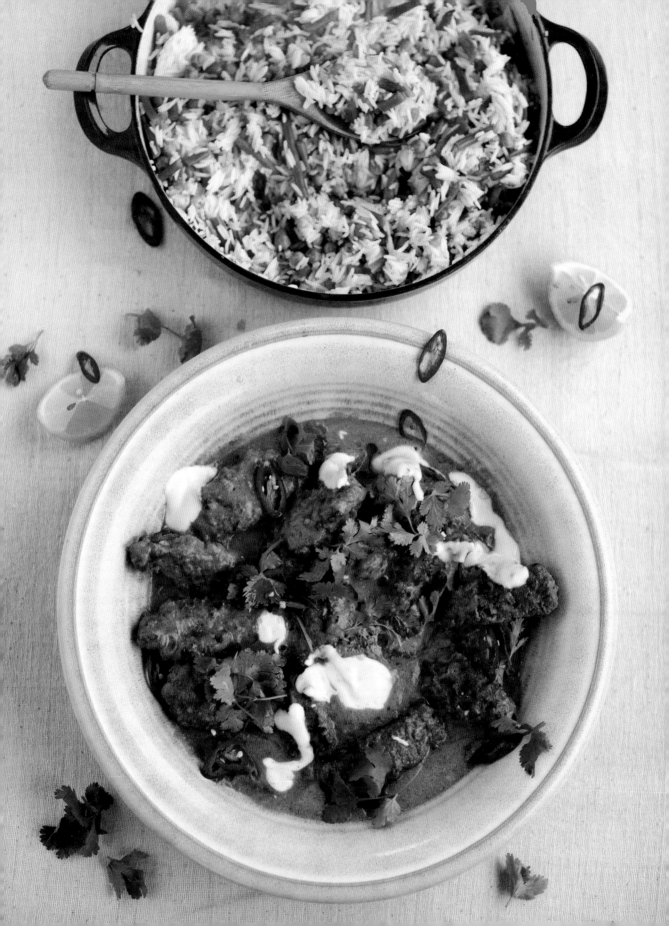

SEARED ASIAN BEEF
BEST NOODLE SALAD & GINGER DRESSING

SERVES 4 | 585 CALORIES

Ingredients out • Kettle boiled • Large frying pan, high heat

Salad
50g cashew nuts
1 tbsp sunflower seeds
2 tbsp sesame seeds
200g fine rice noodles
1 romaine lettuce
1 large carrot
1 bunch of radishes
½ a cucumber
1 big bunch of fresh coriander
3 spring onions
1 punnet of cress
1 pack of alfalfa sprouts

Steak
1 x 450g rump steak, fat removed
2 tsp Chinese five-spice
olive oil

Dressing
1 x 105g pack of pickled ginger
2 limes
1 tbsp fish sauce
1 tbsp low-salt soy sauce
1 tbsp sesame oil
½ a fresh red chilli

START COOKING

Toast the cashews, sunflower and sesame seeds in the frying pan, tossing regularly until golden, then tip into a bowl, return the pan to the heat and turn the heat up to high • Put the noodles into another bowl with a pinch of salt and cover with boiling water • Rub the steak with salt, pepper and the five-spice, and put into the frying pan with 1 tablespoon of olive oil, turning every minute until cooked to your liking

In another bowl, mix together the pickled ginger and its juice, the juice of 1 to 2 limes, the fish and soy sauces and sesame oil, then finely slice and add the chilli • Trim the lettuce and break the leaves apart, shredding any larger ones, then scatter over a large board • Coarsely grate over the trimmed carrot, using a box grater • Halve the radishes, roughly chop the cucumber and the top leafy half of the coriander and trim and finely slice the spring onions

Pile all the veg on the board, snip over the cress and scatter over the alfalfa sprouts • Drain the noodles, rinse and drain again, then add them to the board • When the steak is done, move it to a board to rest, then slice and place on top of the salad, pouring over any resting juices • Scatter over the nuts and serve the dressing on the side, with any remaining lime wedges

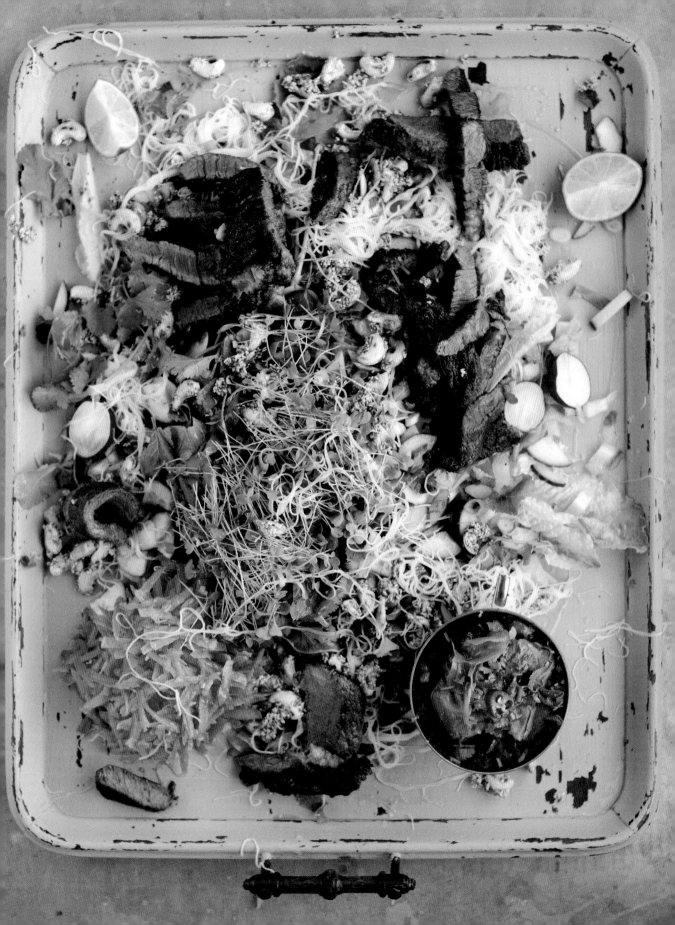

GRILLED STEAK
RATATOUILLE & SAFFRON RICE

SERVES 4 | 593 CALORIES

Ingredients out • Kettle boiled • Griddle pan, high heat • Small lidded pan, medium heat • Shallow lidded casserole pan, medium heat

Ratatouille
1 courgette
1 small aubergine
2 mixed-colour peppers
1 red onion
1 heaped tsp harissa
2 anchovy fillets
2–4 cloves of garlic
700g passata
1 tbsp balsamic vinegar
½ a bunch of fresh basil
2 tbsp fat-free natural yoghurt

Rice
1 mug (300g) of 10-minute
  wholegrain or basmati rice
1 good pinch of saffron
½ a lemon

Steaks
2 x 250g sirloin steaks,
  fat removed
1 tsp sweet paprika
olive oil
½ a bunch of fresh
  flat-leaf parsley
1 heaped tsp Dijon mustard
1 tbsp extra virgin olive oil
½ a lemon

START COOKING

Halve the courgette lengthways, slice the aubergine 1cm thick and place both on the griddle pan, turning when charred • Put 1 mug of rice, 2 mugs of boiling water, the saffron, lemon half and a pinch of salt into the small pan, cover and cook until fluffy, stirring occasionally • Tear the seeds and stalks out of the peppers, then roughly chop with the peeled red onion and put into the casserole pan with the harissa, anchovies and 1 teaspoon of their oil • Squash in the unpeeled garlic through a garlic crusher and stir regularly

Remove the charred courgette and aubergine from the griddle pan, leaving it on the heat, and roughly chop them on a board • Add them to the casserole pan along with the passata and vinegar, and boil with the lid on • Rub the steaks with salt, the paprika and 1 teaspoon of olive oil and place on the hot griddle pan, turning every minute until cooked to your liking

On a board, finely slice the parsley stalks and roughly chop the leaves • Add the mustard and extra virgin olive oil, season with salt and pepper and squeeze over the lemon juice, then mix together and spread over the board • When the steaks are done, transfer them to the board, turn in the dressing, then slice • Tear the top leafy half of the basil into the ratatouille, season to taste, and serve with yoghurt and saffron rice

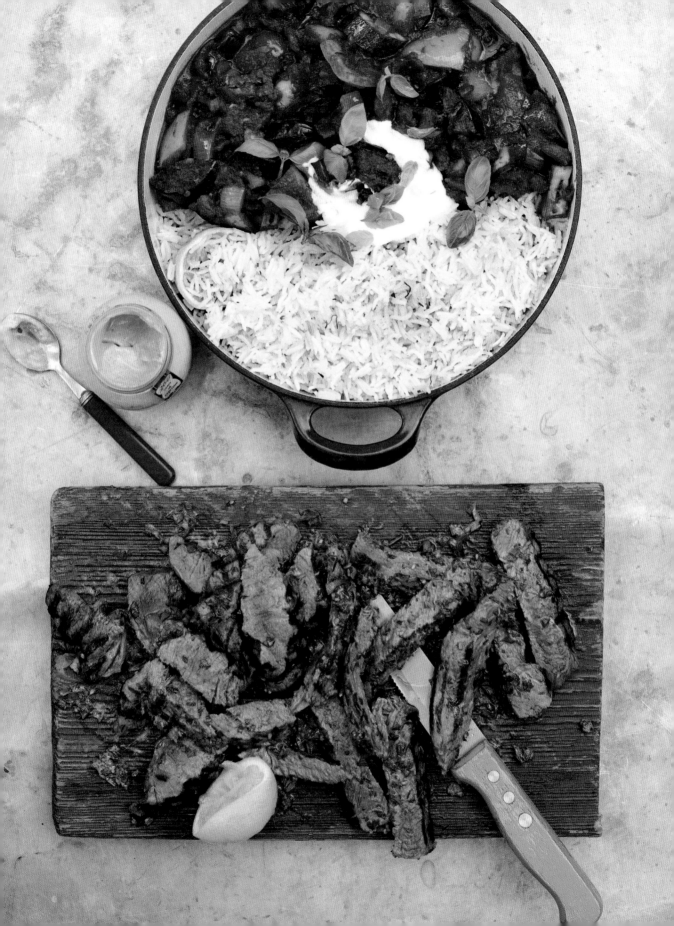

BEEF CHIMICHURRI
NEW POTATOES & CRUNCH SALAD

Ingredients out • Kettle boiled • Medium lidded pan, high heat • Liquidizer • Large frying pan, high heat

Potatoes
800g baby new potatoes
1 lemon
1 tsp dried dill

Beef
4 cloves of garlic
6 spring onions
2 heaped tsp dried oregano
½ a fresh red chilli
1 fresh bay leaf
1 bunch of fresh coriander
2–3 tbsp red wine vinegar
2 x 250g sirloin steaks,
    fat removed
olive oil

Salad
2 little gem lettuces
1 handful of ripe mixed-colour
    tomatoes
½ a bunch of fresh mint
1 punnet of cress
150g popped raw peas
extra virgin olive oil
1 tbsp balsamic vinegar
Parmesan cheese, to serve

START COOKING

Put the new potatoes and whole lemon into the medium pan, then cover with boiling salted water and the lid • Peel the garlic and put into the liquidizer with the trimmed and halved spring onions, the oregano, chilli, bay leaf and coriander (reserving a few leaves) • Add the vinegar and a splash of boiling water, whiz until smooth, season to taste and pour into a bowl

Rub the steaks with salt and pepper, then put into the hot frying pan with 1 tablespoon of olive oil, turning every minute until cooked to your liking • Roughly chop the lettuces, tomatoes and the top leafy half of the mint and place on a platter, then snip over the cress and sprinkle over the raw peas • Dress with 1 tablespoon of extra virgin olive oil and the balsamic, and finish with a grating of Parmesan

Drain the potatoes and lemon, tip into a bowl and use tongs to squash the lemon juice over the potatoes, then discard • Toss with 1 tablespoon of extra virgin olive oil, salt, pepper and the dill, then transfer to the platter • Add the steaks and chimichurri sauce to the platter, sprinkle with the reserved coriander leaves and slice at the table

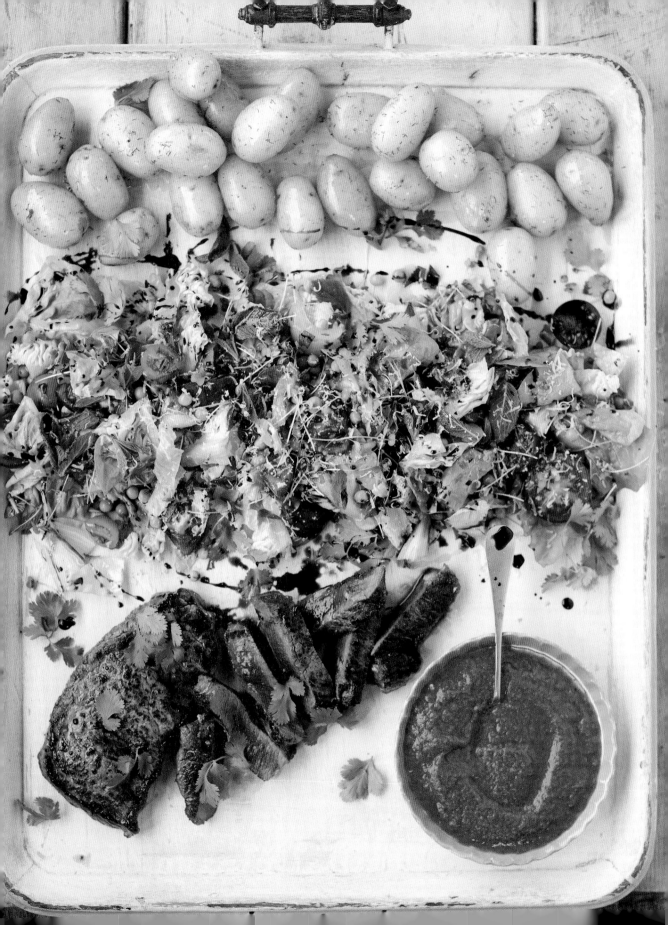

STEAK, LIVER & BACON
BUBBLE & SQUEAK MASH, RED ONION GRAVY

SERVES 4 | 556 CALORIES

Mash
800g potatoes
500g Brussels sprouts
1 splash of semi-skimmed milk

Steak
1 x 300g fillet steak
200g calves' liver slices
1 tbsp English mustard powder
olive oil
4 rashers of smoked streaky bacon
a few sprigs of fresh lemon thyme

Gravy
2 red onions
2 sprigs of fresh rosemary
1 heaped tsp plain flour
1 tbsp blackberry jam
1 tbsp Worcestershire sauce
1 swig of smooth beer or ale
1 chicken stock cube

Ingredients out • Kettle boiled • Food processor (thick slicer) • Large lidded pan, medium heat • Medium frying pan, high heat • Small casserole pan, high heat

START COOKING

Thickly slice the potatoes and Brussels sprouts in the processor, then tip into the large pan and cover with boiling salted water and the lid • Rub the steak and liver slices with salt and the mustard powder • Press and whack the steak out so it's 3cm thick, then add only the steak to the frying pan with 1 tablespoon of oil, turning every minute until cooked to your liking

Peel and halve the onions, then slice them in the processor and tip into the casserole pan with 1 tablespoon of oil and the rosemary leaves, stirring regularly • Drain the veg, return them to the pan, mash with the milk, and season to taste • Stir the flour into the onions, followed by the jam, Worcestershire sauce and beer or ale, crumble in the stock cube and add 300ml of boiling water, then season with salt and pepper and simmer

Remove the steak to a plate to rest, then add the bacon to the pan • When you flip it, add the liver slices and thyme sprigs, turning after a minute or so • Serve the mash on a nice board or platter with the liver, bacon and crispy thyme on top, slice up and add the steak and any resting juices, and serve the gravy in a jug on the side

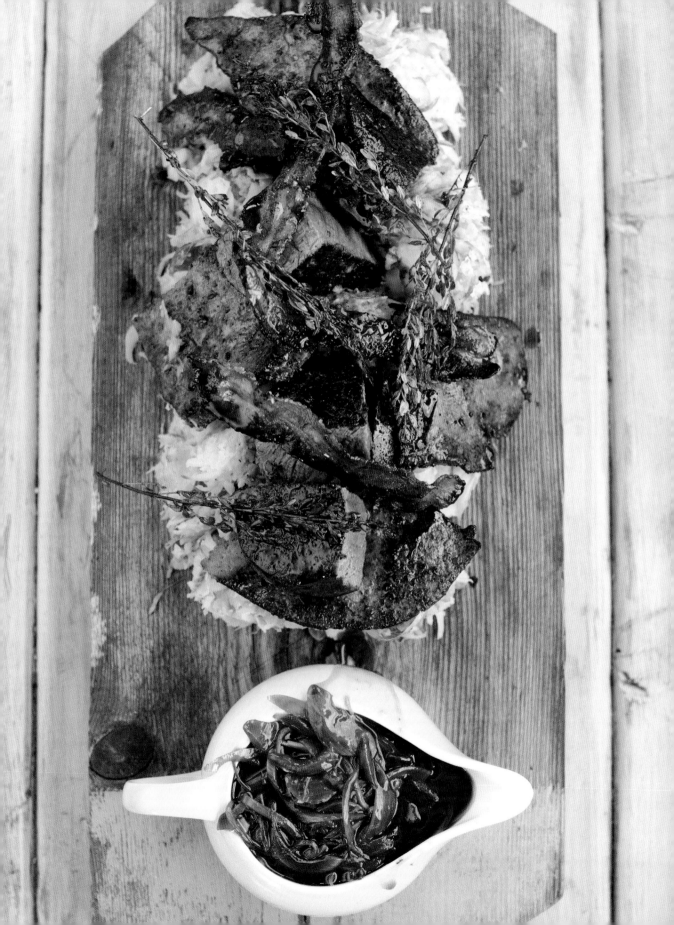

KOREAN FRIED RICE
STEAK, MUSHROOMS & PICKLES

SERVES 4 | 545 CALORIES

Ingredients out • Large frying pan, medium heat
• Griddle pan, high heat • Food processor (fine slicer)

Rice
2 x 250g packs of cooked
   brown rice
1 lemon

Steak & mushrooms
125g oyster mushrooms
sesame oil
low-salt soy sauce
sherry vinegar
1 clove of garlic
2 x 250g sirloin steaks,
   fat removed

Pickle
1 cucumber
2 spring onions
caster sugar

Garnishes
1 little gem lettuce
1 tbsp harissa,
   plus extra to serve
100g baby spinach
2 large eggs
2 tbsp sesame seeds

START COOKING
Tip the cooked rice into the frying pan, squeeze over the lemon juice and stir regularly • Place the mushrooms on the griddle pan, turning when charred • Put 1 tablespoon of oil, 2 tablespoons of soy sauce and 1 tablespoon of sherry vinegar in a medium bowl, squash in the unpeeled garlic through a garlic crusher, then mix well to create a marinade • Slice the steaks 1cm thick

Tip the mushrooms into the bowl of marinade, then lay the steak over the griddle in one layer, cook until nicely charred on one side only, then toss with the mushrooms and marinade • Finely slice the cucumber and trimmed spring onions in the processor, then tip into a bowl • Add a pinch of salt and sugar, and a drizzle of soy sauce and sherry vinegar, then with clean hands scrunch everything together

Shred the lettuce and put in a little bowl, then put the harissa and spinach in similar bowls • Tip the rice into a large bowl • Add 1 teaspoon of oil to the frying pan, crack in the eggs, sprinkle over the sesame seeds, then cook for 1½ minutes on each side so that the yolks are still soft, and place on top of the rice • To serve, mix everything together like a giant salad and adjust the spice to your liking with a little extra harissa

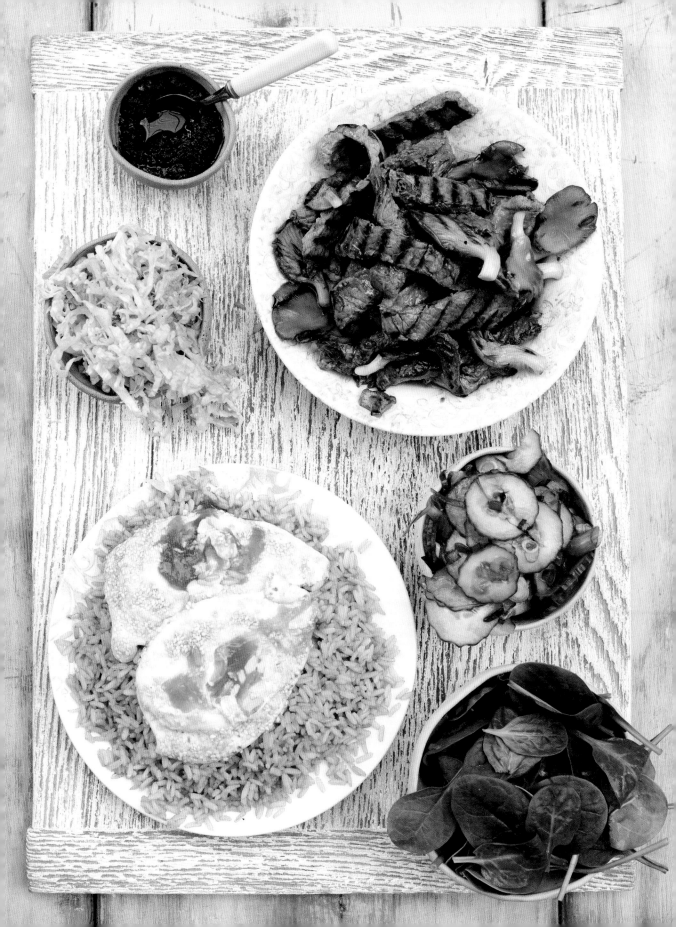

SWEDISH MEATBALLS
CELERIAC & SPINACH RICE

SERVES 4 | 576 CALORIES

Ingredients out • Kettle boiled • Lidded casserole pan, medium heat • Small lidded pan, medium heat • Medium frying pan, medium heat

Rice

1 celeriac

olive oil

a few sprigs of fresh lemon thyme

1 mug (300g) of 10-minute wholegrain or basmati rice

200g baby spinach

Meatballs

200g lean beef mince

200g lean pork mince

½ a bunch of fresh dill

2 tsp caraway seeds

1 swig of vodka

4 tsp cranberry jam

4 tbsp single cream

4 tbsp fat-free natural yoghurt, to serve

START COOKING

Carefully trim the knobbly end off the celeriac, remove the skin, then dice it into 1cm pieces • Put into the casserole pan with 1 tablespoon of oil, a pinch of salt and pepper, the thyme leaves and a splash of boiling water • Put the lid on, turn the heat to high and cook, stirring regularly • Put 1 mug of rice, 2 mugs of boiling water and a pinch of salt into the small pan and put the lid on

Put all the mince into a bowl with a pinch of salt and pepper, finely chop and add most of the dill, then mix and scrunch together with clean hands • Divide the mixture into 4, then pinch and quickly roll out 5 balls from each piece with wet hands • Pour 1 tablespoon of oil into the hot frying pan, add the meatballs and caraway seeds, turn the heat up to high and toss regularly until the meatballs are golden

Stir the spinach into the casserole pan, followed by the cooked rice, then season to taste • Add a good swig of vodka to the meatballs, carefully light it with a match (if you want), let the flames subside, then add the jam, cream and a few good splashes of water, and simmer • Season and serve with the rice, scattered with the remaining dill leaves and yoghurt

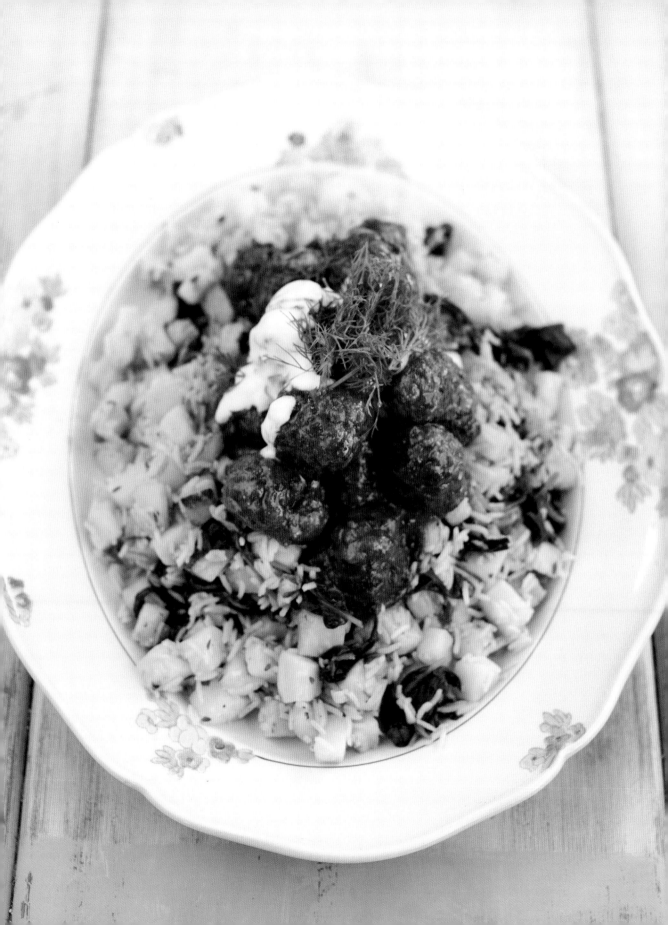

BLACK BEAN BEEF BURGERS NOODLES & PICKLE SALAD

SERVES 4 | 558 CALORIES

Ingredients out • *Kettle boiled* • *Medium frying pan, medium-high heat*
• *Wok, high heat* • *Food processor (fine slicer)*

Burgers

400g lean beef mince
6 tbsp black bean sauce
olive oil
1 tbsp runny honey
2 tbsp sesame seeds
1 lime

Noodles

1 chicken stock cube
1 thumb-sized piece of ginger
4 nests of egg noodles
2 mixed-colour peppers
200g sugar snap peas
2 bok choi
150g mixed mushrooms
1 lime

Salad

1 x 225g tin of water chestnuts
3 spring onions
½ a fresh red chilli
1 lime
½ a bunch of fresh coriander
low-salt soy sauce

START COOKING

Put the mince, half the black bean sauce and a pinch of salt and pepper into a bowl and scrunch together with your hands • Divide the mixture into 4 pieces and shape each one into a patty about 2cm thick with wet hands • Put into the frying pan with 1 tablespoon of oil, turning when golden • Pour 600ml of boiling water into the wok, crumble in the stock cube, then peel, slice and add the ginger

Drain the water chestnuts and slice in the processor with the trimmed spring onions and chilli, then tip into a bowl • Add the juice of 1 lime and a pinch of salt, then scrunch and toss together • Rip off and add the top leafy half of the coriander (reserving the stalks) and drizzle with a little soy, then put aside • Put the noodles into the wok to boil for 2 minutes, breaking them apart, then add the rest of the black bean sauce and the juice from 1 lime

Rip the seeds and stalks out of the peppers, then slice in the processor with the sugar snaps, bok choi and coriander stalks • Tip the sliced veg into the wok, tear in the mushrooms and cook for 1 minute, then serve in a nice bowl • Sprinkle the burgers with the honey and sesame seeds and toss to coat, then transfer them to a serving board with lime wedges and the pickle salad, tossing the pickle at the last minute

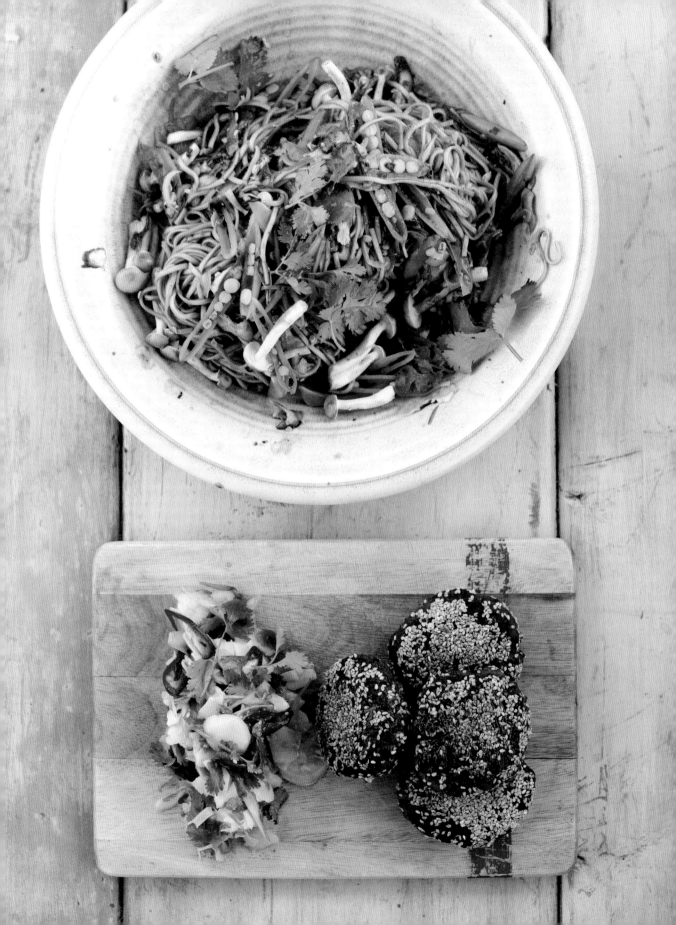

STEAK MEDALLIONS
MUSHROOM SAUCE & SPRING GREENS

SERVES 4 | 445 CALORIES

Ingredients out • Kettle boiled • Casserole pan, high heat • Medium frying pan, medium heat • Griddle pan, high heat • Stick blender

Mushroom sauce
30g dried porcini mushrooms
olive oil
250g mixed mushrooms
2 cloves of garlic
1 good splash of brandy
4 tbsp single cream
1 tsp truffle oil

Greens
800g baby new potatoes
½ a savoy cabbage (roughly 400g)
200g tenderstem broccoli
250g frozen peas
1 tbsp extra virgin olive oil
½ a lemon

Steak
4 x 125g fillet steak medallions
150g oyster mushrooms

START COOKING

Put the porcini into a mug and cover with boiling water • Halving any larger ones, put the new potatoes into the casserole pan and cover with boiling salted water and the lid • Slice the cabbage 2.5cm thick, add it to the pan and replace the lid • Put 1 tablespoon of olive oil into the frying pan and tear in the mixed mushrooms • Squash the unpeeled garlic through a garlic crusher over the top, add the porcini (reserving the liquid) and a pinch of salt and pepper, and toss regularly

Rub the steaks with salt, pepper and 1 tablespoon of olive oil, then place on the griddle pan with the oyster mushrooms, turning the steaks every minute until cooked to your liking • Trim the ends off the broccoli, then add it to the casserole pan with the peas to cook for 2 minutes • Drain, toss in the extra virgin olive oil and the juice of ½ a lemon, and season to taste

Add the brandy to the mixed mushrooms, carefully light it with a match (if you want), let the flames subside, then add the cream and truffle oil and bring to the boil • Adjust the consistency with the reserved porcini liquid (discarding any gritty bits), then blend the sauce to the consistency of your liking and season to taste • Serve with the steaks, oyster mushrooms, spuds and greens

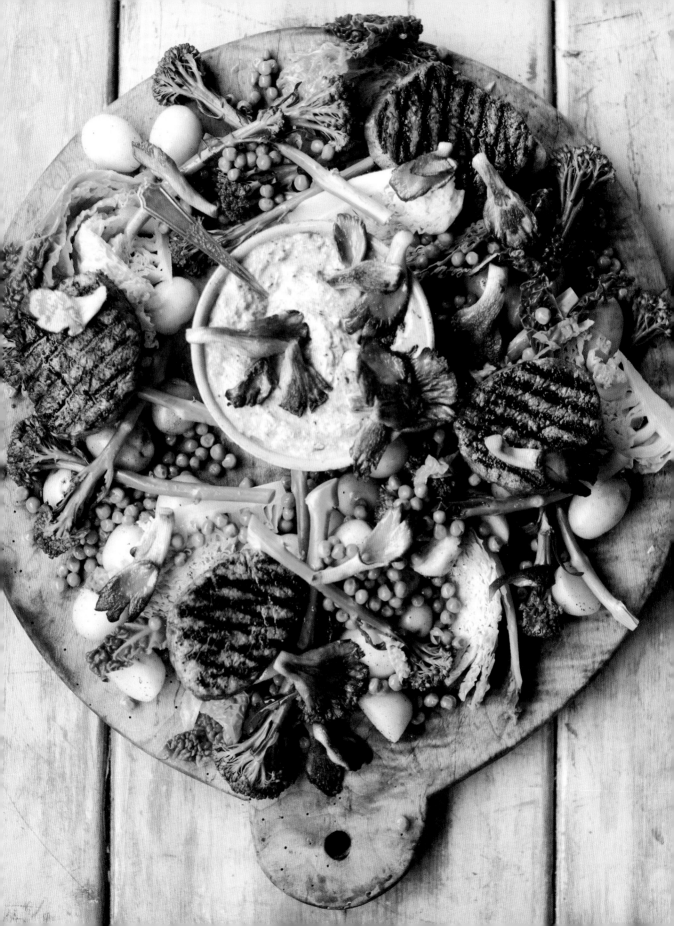

CAJUN STEAK
SMOKY BAKED BEANS & COLLARD GREENS

Greens

2 rashers of smoked pancetta
olive oil
1 big bunch of mixed fresh herbs,
    such as bay, thyme and rosemary
1 carrot
4 spring onions
½ a bunch of radishes
200g curly kale
1 chicken stock cube

Beans

2 x 400g tins of mixed beans
350g passata
1 tsp Worcestershire sauce
1 tsp Tabasco
2 tbsp tomato ketchup
2 tbsp HP sauce
1 tsp runny honey
1 heaped tsp English mustard,
    plus extra to serve
40g Cheddar cheese

Steak

2 x 250g sirloin steaks, fat removed
1 tsp sweet paprika
1 tsp dried thyme

Chilli vinegar

1 fresh red chilli
1 bottle of white wine vinegar

Ingredients out • Kettle boiled • Oven at full whack (240°C/475°F/gas 9) • Large lidded pan, medium-high heat • Medium ovenproof frying pan, medium heat • Large frying pan, high heat

START COOKING

Slice the pancetta, put it into the lidded pan with 1 tablespoon of oil, then pick in the herb leaves • Trim, finely slice and add the carrot, spring onions and radishes, stirring regularly • Drain and rinse the beans and put into the medium frying pan with 2 tablespoons of oil to fry and crisp up

Slice the kale (if needed) and add to the lidded pan, crumble in the stock cube and pour over 300ml of boiling water, then put the lid on • Stir the remaining beans ingredients (except the cheese) into the beans pan and bring to the boil • Grate over the Cheddar, then place in the oven until golden and sizzling

Rub the steaks with salt, pepper, the paprika and thyme • Put them into the really hot large frying pan with 1 tablespoon of oil, turning every minute until cooked to your liking • Slice the chilli and add to the bottle of vinegar with a couple of bay leaves, if you have them (it will keep for months), then add a drizzle to the greens before serving • Carve the steaks on a board at the table and serve with the beans, greens and a splodge of mustard

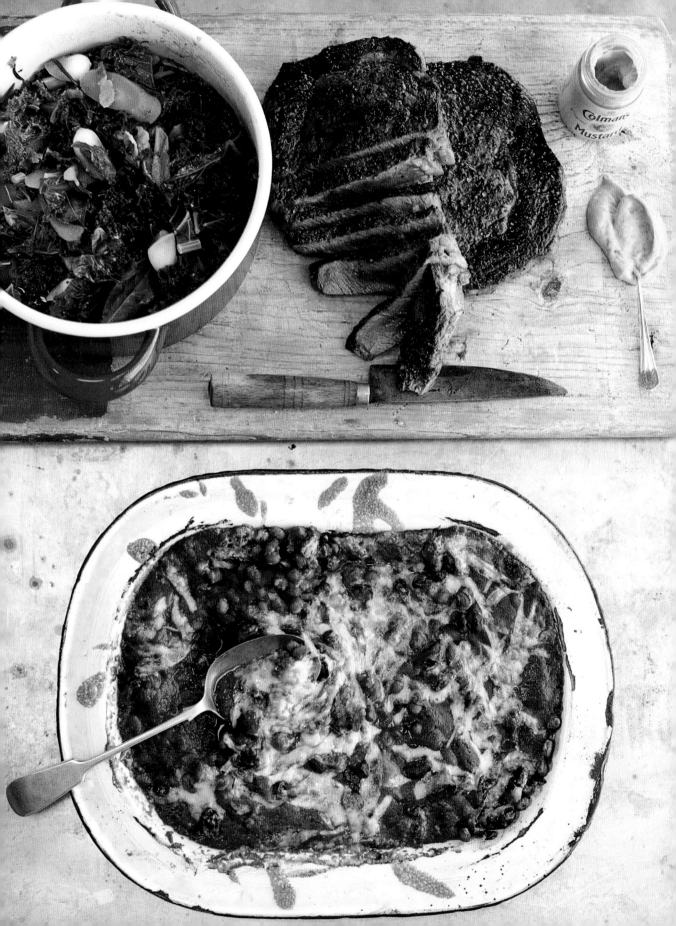

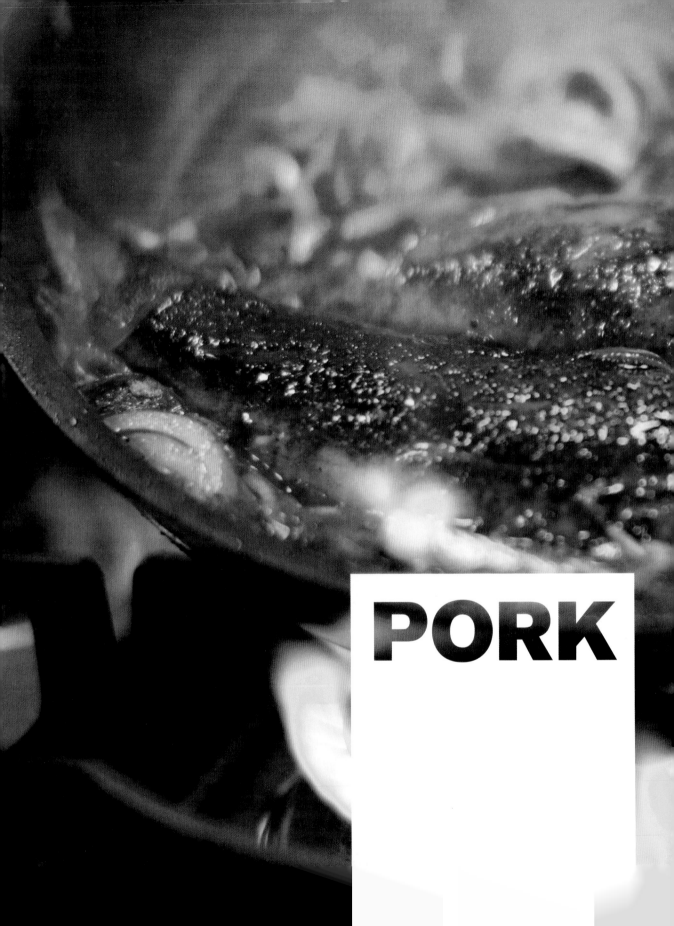

PORK

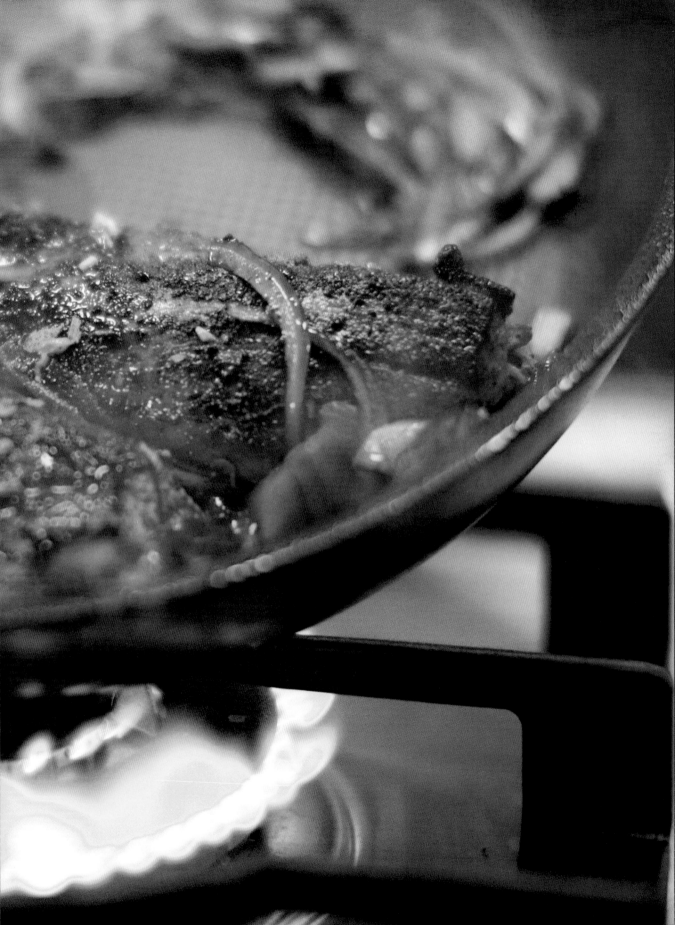

CRISPY PARMA PORK
MINTED COURGETTES & BROWN RICE

SERVES 4 | 582 CALORIES

Ingredients out • Large frying pan, medium heat
• Food processor (fine slicer) • Large casserole pan, medium heat

Pork

400g pork fillet
40g feta cheese
4 slices of Parma ham
olive oil
8 fresh sage leaves
balsamic vinegar

Courgettes

6 medium mixed-colour courgettes
5 cloves of garlic
1 fresh red chilli
½ a bunch of fresh mint

To serve

2 tsp sun-dried tomato paste
1 lemon
2 x 250g packs of cooked
   brown rice
4 tbsp fat-free natural yoghurt

START COOKING

Cut the pork into 8 even-sized medallions and make a slit in the centre of each one • Cut the feta into 8 pieces and poke these into the slits in the pork, then sprinkle with a little black pepper and wrap each piece with ½ a slice of Parma ham • Flatten with your fist and put into the frying pan, ham side down, with 1 tablespoon of oil, turning regularly until golden and cooked through

Finely slice the courgettes in the processor and add to the casserole pan with 2 tablespoons of oil • Squash in the unpeeled garlic through a garlic crusher and turn the heat up to high • Finely chop the chilli and most of the top leafy half of the mint and add to the pan, season to taste with salt and pepper, then stir regularly until softened and delicious

Add the sage leaves to the pork pan for 30 seconds until crispy • Tip the courgettes on to a serving platter and arrange the pork and sage on top • Return the frying pan to a high heat, add a splash of water, the sun-dried tomato paste and lemon juice, then tip in the rice and warm through for 1 minute • Serve the rice drizzled with yoghurt, drizzle a little balsamic over the pork, then scatter everything with the remaining mint leaves

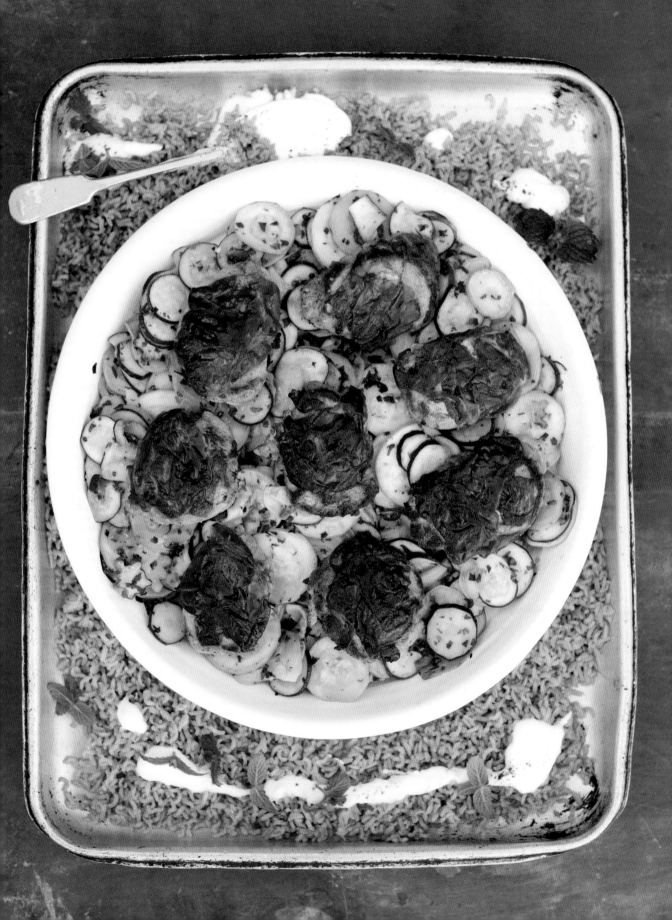

GLAZED PORK FILLET
CAJUN-STYLE PEPPER RICE & BBQ SAUCE

SERVES 4 | 611 CALORIES

Ingredients out • *Oven grill on medium-high* • *Large frying pan, medium heat*
• *Large casserole pan, high heat*

Pork
600g pork fillet
1 heaped tsp ground allspice
olive oil

Rice
1 red onion
1 stick of celery
175g okra
2 mixed-colour peppers
1 tsp sweet smoked paprika
1 pinch of cumin seeds
1 tsp fennel seeds
2 x 250g packs of cooked
    brown rice
1 lemon
½ a bunch of fresh basil

BBQ sauce
2 cloves of garlic
2 tbsp Worcestershire sauce
4 heaped tbsp tomato ketchup
2 tbsp HP sauce
1 heaped tbsp runny honey
1 tbsp low-salt soy sauce
1 tsp Tabasco
3 tbsp fresh apple juice

To serve
pickled veg
4 tbsp fat-free natural yoghurt

START COOKING

Score lengthways halfway through the centre of the pork, open it out like a book, then flatten it slightly with your fist • Rub with salt, pepper and the allspice, then put it into the frying pan with 1 tablespoon of oil, turning when it has a dark golden crust (roughly 4 minutes) • Roughly chop the peeled onion, trimmed celery, okra, and deseeded peppers, putting them into the casserole pan as you go with 1 tablespoon of oil, then add the paprika, cumin and fennel seeds and a cup of water, stirring regularly

Squash the unpeeled garlic through a garlic crusher into a bowl, add all the remaining sauce ingredients and a pinch of salt, then mix well • When the pork has a good crust on both sides, transfer to a baking dish • Pour over most of the sauce and place under the grill until the pork is cooked through • Pour the rest of the sauce into a small bowl to serve on the side

Stir the rice into the veg pan, squeeze in the lemon juice, then roughly chop and add the top leafy half of the basil and season to taste • Slice up the glazed pork at the table and serve with the extra sauce and pots of pickled veg such as gherkins, cauliflower, red cabbage and anything else crunchy and delicious • Dollop yoghurt over the rice before serving

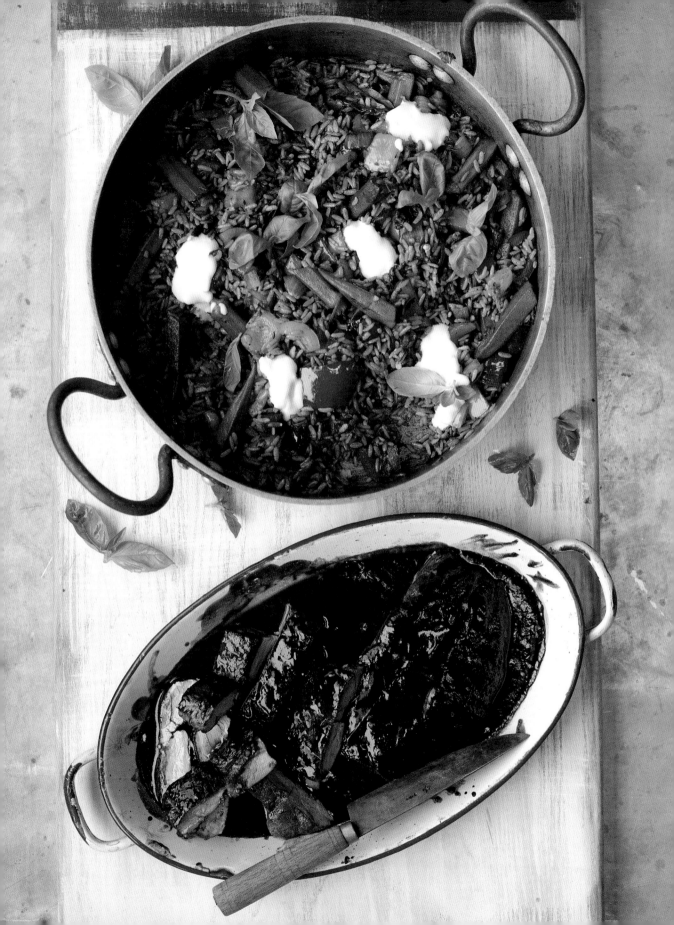

ULTIMATE PORK TACOS
SPICY BLACK BEANS & AVOCADO GARDEN SALAD

Ingredients out • *Large frying pan, medium-high heat*
• *Medium frying pan, medium heat*

Pork
350g skinless pork belly
1 heaped tsp fennel seeds
1 heaped tsp sweet smoked
   paprika

Beans
olive oil
1 good pinch of cumin seeds
3 spring onions
2 cloves of garlic
1 x 400g tin of black beans

Salad
1 fresh red or green chilli
2 little gem lettuces
½ a bunch of fresh coriander
1 ripe avocado
1 large ripe tomato
1 eating apple
low-salt soy sauce
1 tbsp extra virgin olive oil
1 lime

To serve
Lingham's chilli sauce
4 tbsp fat-free natural yoghurt
8 corn taco shells

START COOKING

Cut the pork into 1cm dice and tip into the large frying pan with the fennel seeds, paprika, salt and pepper, and stir regularly • Put 1 tablespoon of olive oil and the cumin seeds into the medium frying pan • Trim, slice and add the spring onions, squash in the unpeeled garlic through a garlic crusher, then stir in the beans and their juices, and simmer

Finely slice the chilli, lettuce and most of the top leafy half of the coriander, then halve, destone, peel and chop the avocado, along with the tomato • Toss and pile all this on a platter, coarsely grating or matchsticking the apple on top • Ripple a little chilli sauce through the yoghurt in a small bowl

Stir, mush and season the beans to taste • Drizzle the salad with a little soy sauce, the extra virgin olive oil and lime juice, then toss together • Drain the fat from the pork pan, then serve everything straight away, with a pile of taco shells and all the other elements, sprinkled with the remaining coriander leaves

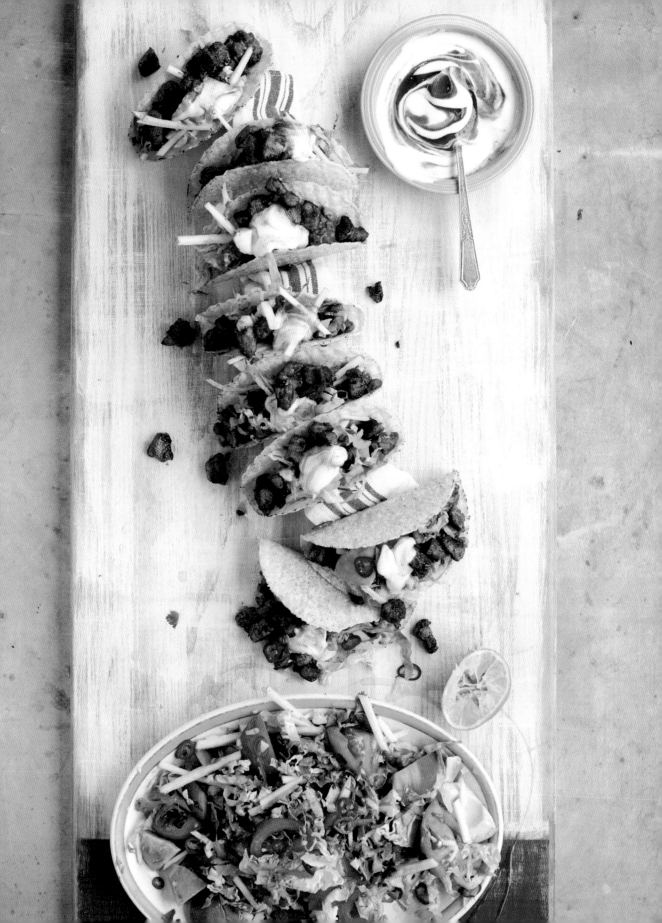

PORK STEAKS
HUNGARIAN PEPPER SAUCE & RICE

SERVES 4 | 685 CALORIES

Ingredients out • Kettle boiled • Food processor (thick slicer) • Large casserole pan, medium heat • Medium lidded pan, medium heat • Griddle pan, high heat

Sauce
2 mixed-colour peppers
1 red onion
1 carrot
1 bulb of fennel
1 eating apple
olive oil
2 tsp sweet smoked paprika,
    plus extra to serve
4–5 fresh bay leaves
4 cloves of garlic
2 tbsp balsamic vinegar
700g passata

Pork
500g pork fillet
1 tsp ground coriander

To serve
1 mug (300g) of 10-minute
    wholegrain or basmati rice
70g rocket
1 lemon
4 tbsp fat-free natural yoghurt

START COOKING

Deseed the peppers, peel and halve the onion, trim the carrot, trim and quarter the fennel (reserving any leafy tops), then slice them all in the processor with the apple • Put 2 tablespoons of oil into the casserole pan, tip in the sliced veg, add the paprika and bay leaves, squash in the unpeeled garlic through a garlic crusher, season with salt and pepper, and fry, stirring regularly

Put 1 mug of rice and 2 mugs of boiling water into the medium pan with a good pinch of salt, cover and stir occasionally • Slice the pork into 8 medallions, flatten them slightly with your fist, then rub with salt, pepper, the ground coriander and 1 teaspoon of oil, then put on the griddle pan until cooked through, turning when nicely charred

Add the balsamic and passata to the peppers, season to taste and bring to the boil • Sprinkle the rice with an extra dusting of paprika • Dress the rocket in the bag with the lemon juice and a small pinch of salt, then fold most of it through the sauce • Tip the sauce on to a platter, place the charred pork on top and scatter with the remaining rocket • Drizzle with the yoghurt, scatter over any reserved fennel tops and serve with the fluffy rice

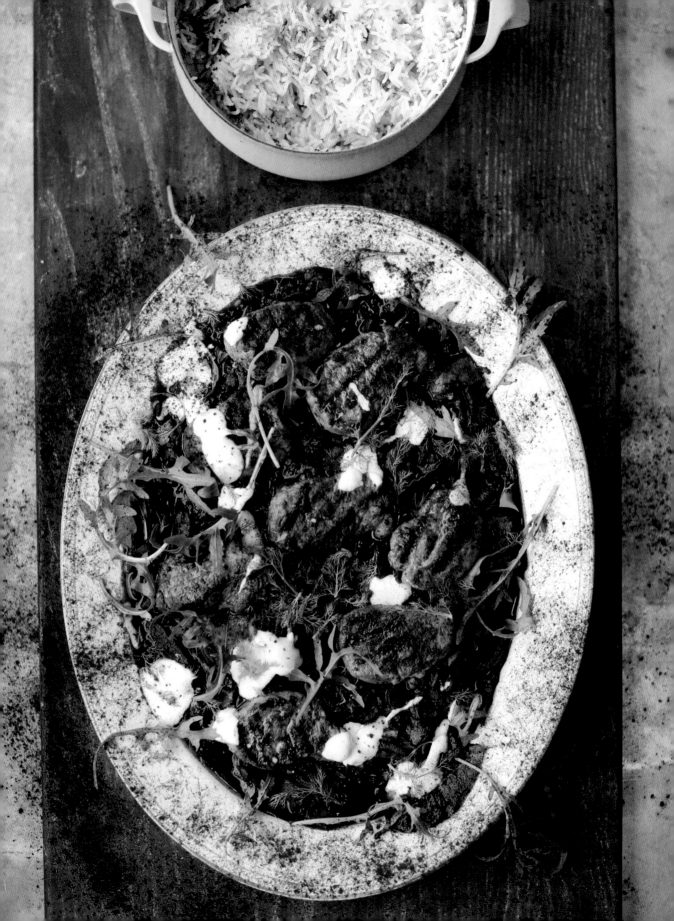

JERK PORK

GRILLED CORN & CRUNCHY TORTILLA SALAD

SERVES 4 | 641 CALORIES

Ingredients out • Oven at 180°C/350°F/gas 4 • Griddle pan, high heat • Large frying pan, high heat • Liquidizer

Salad

4 corn on the cob
8 small corn tortillas
1 romaine lettuce
2 punnets of cress
1 handful of ripe mixed-colour
  cherry tomatoes
1 ripe avocado
1 lime
1 tbsp extra virgin olive oil

Jerk pork

500g pork fillet
1 tsp ground coriander
olive oil
4 spring onions
1 bunch of fresh coriander
2 cloves of garlic
1 thumb-sized piece of ginger
1 heaped tbsp runny honey
½ a Scotch bonnet chilli
  (or milder, if you prefer)
2 fresh bay leaves
1 tsp allspice
1 tbsp low-salt soy sauce
2 tbsp red wine vinegar
6 ripe medium tomatoes

To serve

4 tbsp fat-free natural yoghurt

START COOKING

Put the corn on the griddle pan, turning when charred • Arrange the tortillas around a large heatproof bowl and put into the oven to crisp up for 6 minutes • Cut the pork into 8 medallions, flatten them slightly with your fist, then rub with salt, pepper and the ground coriander, and put into the frying pan with 1 tablespoon of olive oil, turning regularly until golden and cooked through

Put the trimmed spring onions, most of the fresh coriander, the peeled garlic and ginger and the rest of the jerk pork ingredients into the liquidizer with a splash of water and whiz until smooth • Remove the pork from the pan, pour in the jerk sauce and let it boil, then return the pork to the pan and reduce to a simmer • Trim the lettuce and break the leaves apart, then arrange them in the tortilla bowl • Carefully hold the charred corn steady and run a knife down the sides to cut off the kernels, then add them to the bowl

Snip the cress into the bowl, roughly chop and add the cherry tomatoes and peeled, destoned avocado, then gently mix together • Squeeze over the lime juice, add the extra virgin olive oil and a pinch of salt and pepper • Serve the pork and sauce scattered with the remaining coriander leaves and dollops of yoghurt, with the tortilla salad on the side (the salad is really nice dressed with some of the hot sauce)

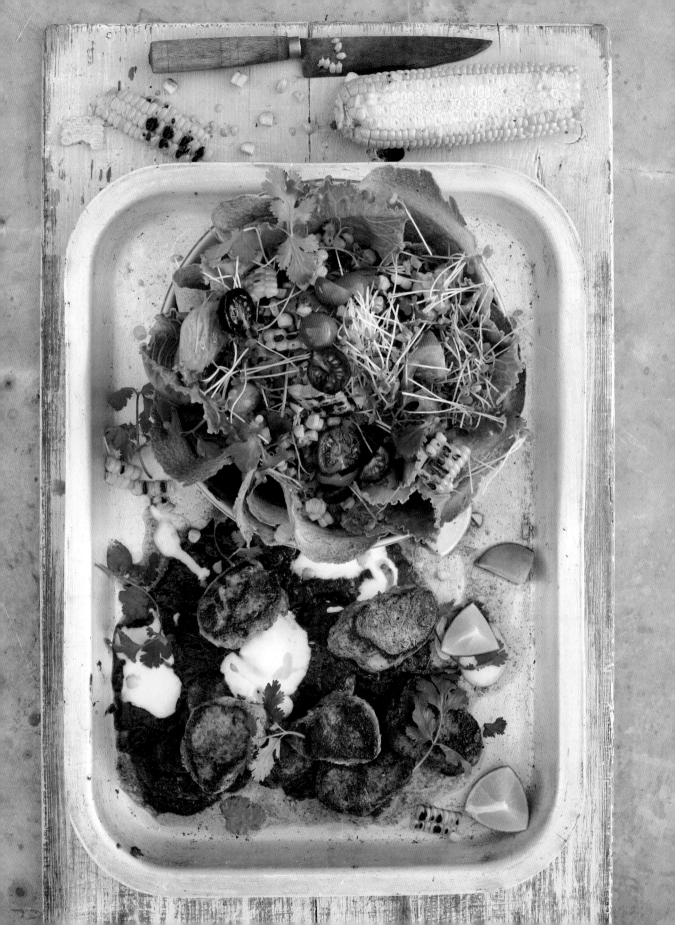

PORK MARSALA
PORCINI RICE & SPRING GREENS

SERVES 4 | 574 CALORIES

Ingredients out • Kettle boiled • Medium lidded casserole pan, medium heat • Large frying pan, high heat • Medium lidded pan, medium heat

Rice

1 mug (300g) of 10-minute
  wholegrain or basmati rice
1 big pinch of dried porcini
  mushrooms
½ a lemon
a few sprigs of fresh lemon thyme

Pork

500g pork fillet
1 heaped tsp ground coriander
1 heaped tsp sweet paprika
olive oil
1 small red onion
a few sprigs of fresh sage
1 swig of Marsala
70ml single cream, plus
  extra to serve

Greens

1 small savoy cabbage
1 chicken stock cube
100g Swiss chard or any other
  dark spring greens
½ a lemon
1 tbsp extra virgin olive oil

START COOKING

Put 1 mug of rice and 2 mugs of boiling water into the casserole pan, tear in the porcini, add a pinch of salt, the lemon half and lemon thyme, then put the lid on • Refill and boil the kettle • Score lengthways halfway through the centre of the pork, open it out like a book, then flatten it slightly with your fist • Rub with salt, pepper, the ground coriander and paprika then, put it into the frying pan with 1 tablespoon of olive oil, turning regularly until golden and cooked through

Click off and trim the outer leaves of the cabbage, then roll them up like a cigar and finely slice them • Cut the inner cabbage into thin wedges, then add all the cabbage to the medium lidded pan, crumble in the stock cube and cover with boiling water • Finely chop the peeled red onion, pick the sage leaves, then add both to the pork to fry for a few minutes • Add the Swiss chard to the cabbage pan and cover • Once the pork is cooked through, add a good swig of Marsala, carefully light it with a match (if you want) and let the flames subside

Transfer the pork to a board, then pour the single cream into the pan and add a ladle or two of stock from the greens, boil and reduce to a nice consistency • Squeeze the juice from the remaining lemon half over the greens, drizzle with the extra virgin olive oil and stir well • Fluff up the rice, carve the pork into 1cm slices, spoon over the sauce and serve with the greens on the side • Drizzle 1 teaspoon of cream over the pork to finish, if you like

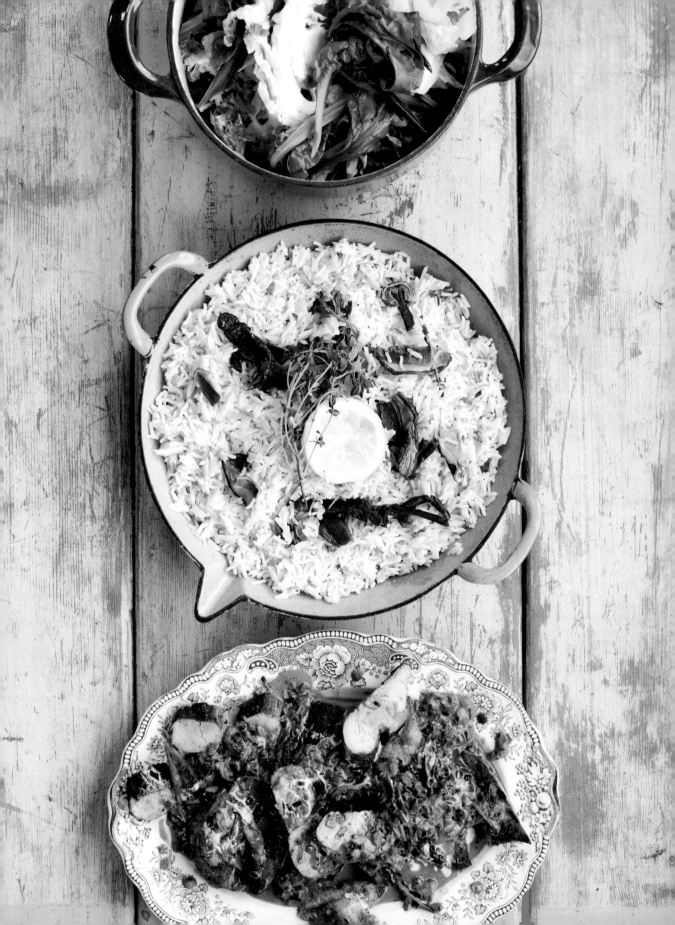

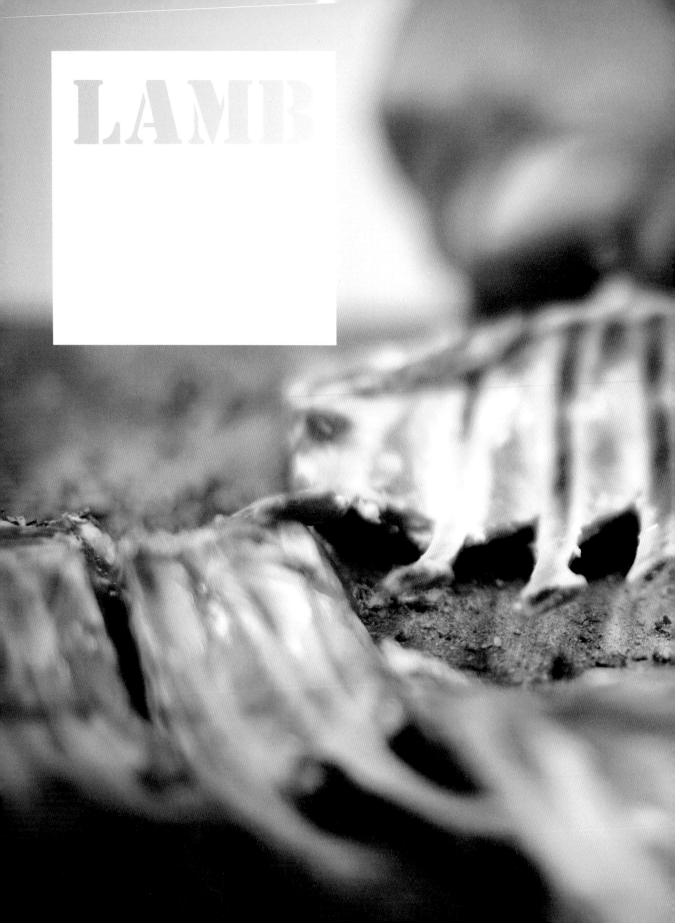

LAMB

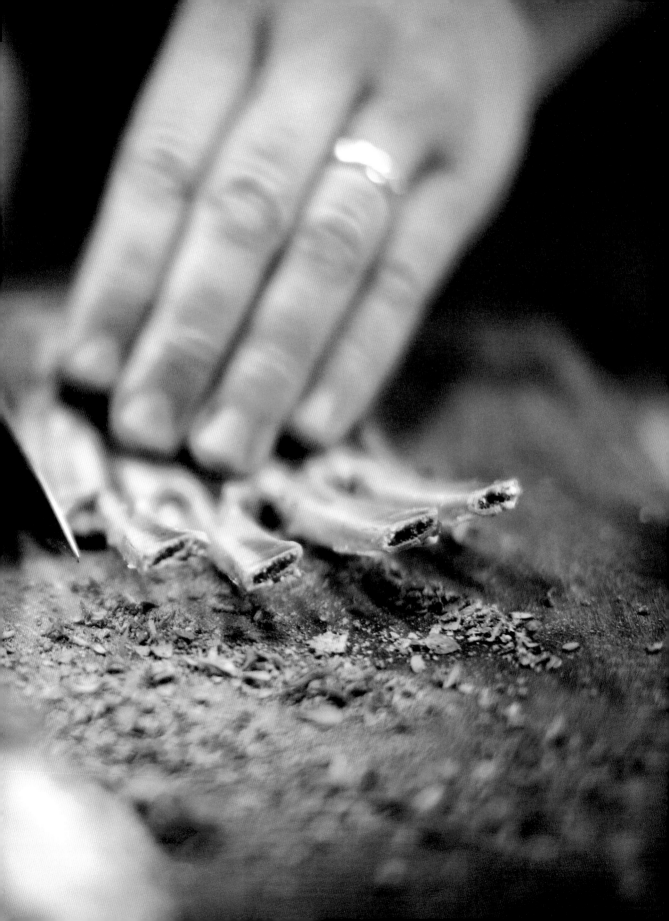

LAMB LOLLIPOPS
CURRY SAUCE, RICE & PEAS

SERVES 4 | 632 CALORIES

Ingredients out • Kettle boiled • Medium lidded pan, high heat
• Two large non-stick frying pans, medium-high heat

Rice & peas
1 mug (300g) of 10-minute
  wholegrain or basmati rice
8 cloves
40g dried red split lentils
300g podded raw or garden peas

Lamb
8 large lamb cutlets on the bone,
  trimmed of fat
1 tbsp garam masala
olive oil
4 spring onions
1 fresh red chilli
1 thumb-sized piece of ginger
4 jarred red peppers
1 heaped tsp runny honey
balsamic vinegar
3 sprigs of fresh coriander

Curry sauce
2 tbsp Patak's korma paste
1 x 400g tin of light coconut milk
1 lemon

Garnishes
2 uncooked poppadoms
fat-free natural yoghurt

START COOKING

Put 1 mug of rice and 2 mugs of boiling water into the medium pan with a pinch of salt and the cloves, then put the lid on, stirring occasionally • Rub the lamb with salt, pepper and the garam masala, bash and flatten them with your fist, then put into one of the hot frying pans with 1 tablespoon of oil, turning when gnarly and golden brown

Put the korma paste and coconut milk into the other frying pan with the juice of ½ a lemon, stir together, bring to the boil and simmer for 5 minutes, then turn the heat off • Mix the lentils into the rice • Trim and slice the spring onions, chilli, peeled ginger and peppers, then toss in with the lamb • Stir the peas into the rice and lentils

Pour half the curry sauce into a bowl (pop the rest in the fridge to use another day) • Break up the uncooked poppadoms and pop in the microwave (800W) for a minute or two to puff up • At the last minute, toss the lamb with the honey and a splash of balsamic • Serve the lamb scattered with coriander leaves and scrunched-up poppadoms, with the rice and peas, yoghurt and lemon wedges on the side

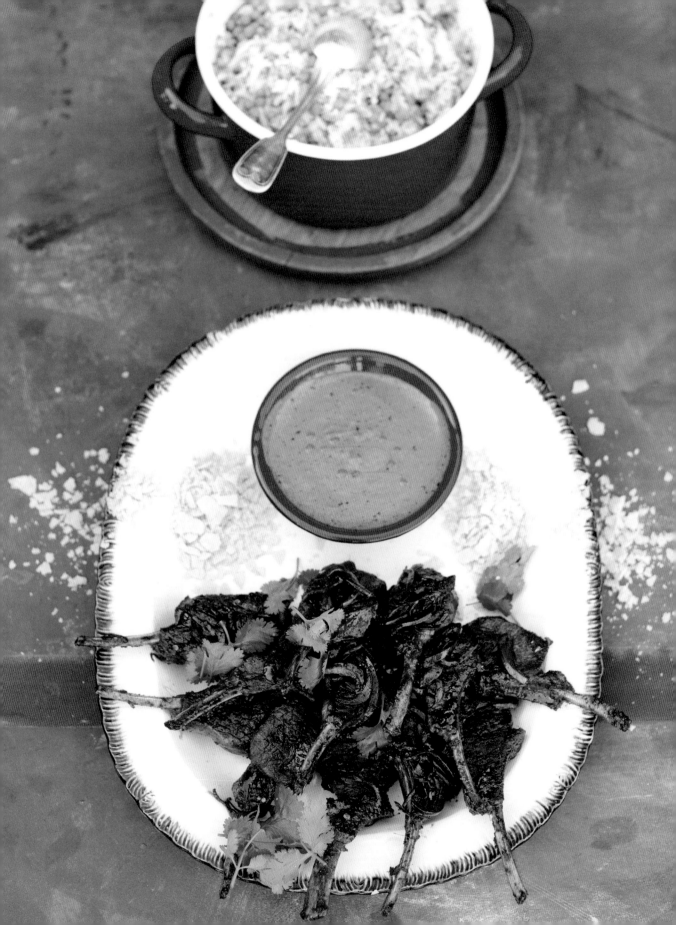

LAMB MEATBALLS
CHOP SALAD & HARISSA YOGHURT

Ingredients out • Kettle boiled • Large frying pan, medium heat
• Large lidded pan, medium-high heat

Meatballs

400g lean lamb mince
1 heaped tsp garam masala
olive oil
1 pinch of saffron
½–1 fresh red chilli
2 spring onions
½ a bunch of fresh coriander
2 cloves of garlic
1 x 400g tin of chickpeas
350g passata

Salad

½ a cucumber
2 little gem lettuces
1 bunch of radishes
2 ripe tomatoes
1 tbsp extra virgin olive oil
1 lemon

To serve

1 heaped tsp harissa
4 heaped tbsp fat-free
   natural yoghurt
8 small wholewheat tortillas
1 orange

START COOKING

Mix the mince in a bowl with salt, pepper and the garam masala • Divide into 4, then roll each piece into 4 balls with wet hands, placing them in the frying pan as you roll them and adding 1 tablespoon of olive oil • Toss regularly until dark golden all over • Put the saffron into a cup, just cover with boiling water and leave to soak

Finely slice the chilli, trimmed spring onions and coriander stalks (reserving the leaves), put them into the large pan with 1 tablespoon of olive oil, then squash in the unpeeled garlic through a garlic crusher • Fry for 40 seconds, then add the saffron and its soaking water, the drained chickpeas and the passata, cover and bring to the boil • In a small dish, swirl the harissa through the yoghurt

Roughly chop and mix all the salad veg for the salad on a board • Add the extra virgin olive oil and lemon juice, then season to taste • Loosen the sauce with a splash of water if needed, then pour into the meatball pan and season to taste • Microwave (800W) the tortillas for 45 seconds • Serve it all with orange wedges and a scattering of coriander leaves

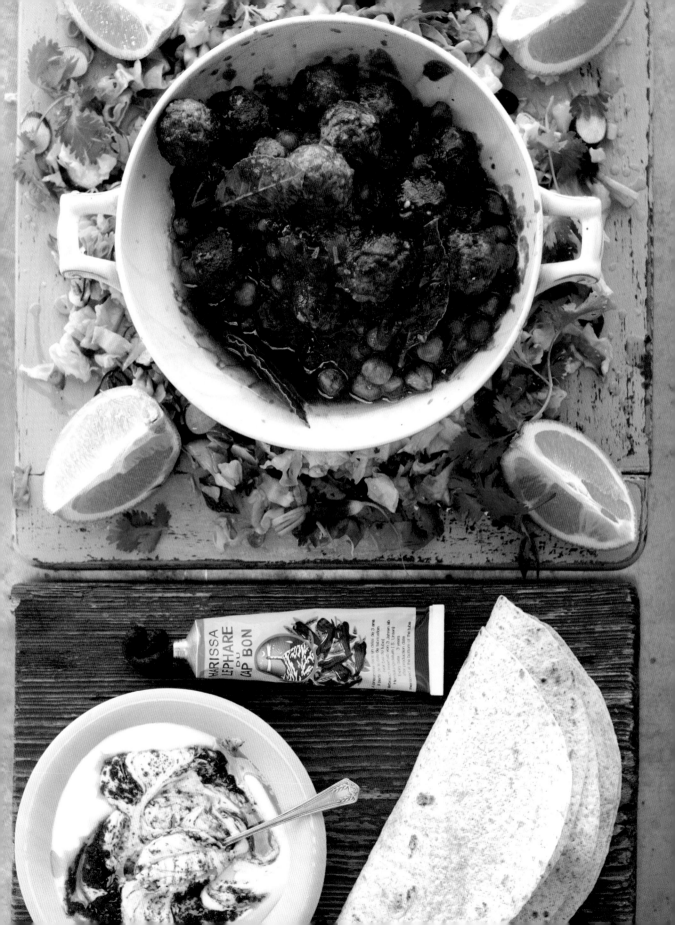

GLAZED SIZZLING CHOPS
SWEET TOMATO & ASPARAGUS LASAGNETTI

Ingredients out • Kettle boiled • Large frying pan, high heat
• Large casserole pan, medium heat

Lamb

8 large lamb chops, trimmed of fat
olive oil
a few sprigs of fresh rosemary
1 tbsp runny honey
2 tbsp balsamic vinegar,
   plus extra to serve

Lasagnetti

4 spring onions
2 bunches of asparagus (600g)
1 fresh red chilli
300g ripe cherry tomatoes
1 bunch of fresh mint
1 small bulb of garlic
300g fresh lasagne sheets
30g Parmesan cheese

START COOKING

Toss the lamb chops with a pinch of salt and put into the frying pan with 1 tablespoon of oil, turning regularly until golden (around 8 minutes) • Trim and finely slice the spring onions, asparagus (leaving the tips whole) and chilli, and halve the cherry tomatoes • Scrape the veg into the casserole pan with 2 tablespoons of oil

Roughly chop most of the top leafy half of the mint and add to the veg with a pinch of salt and pepper, then squash in 3 cloves of unpeeled garlic through a garlic crusher • Bash the remaining unpeeled garlic cloves and add to the lamb with the rosemary leaves • Cut the lasagne sheets into 2cm-thick strips, scatter them over the veg, then cover with 500ml of boiling water and mix together

Reduce the heat under the lamb to low and toss with the honey and balsamic to glaze, then remove to a plate to rest • Finely grate the Parmesan over the lasagnetti and turn the heat off • Serve with the lamb, adding an extra drizzle of balsamic and sprinkling over the remaining mint

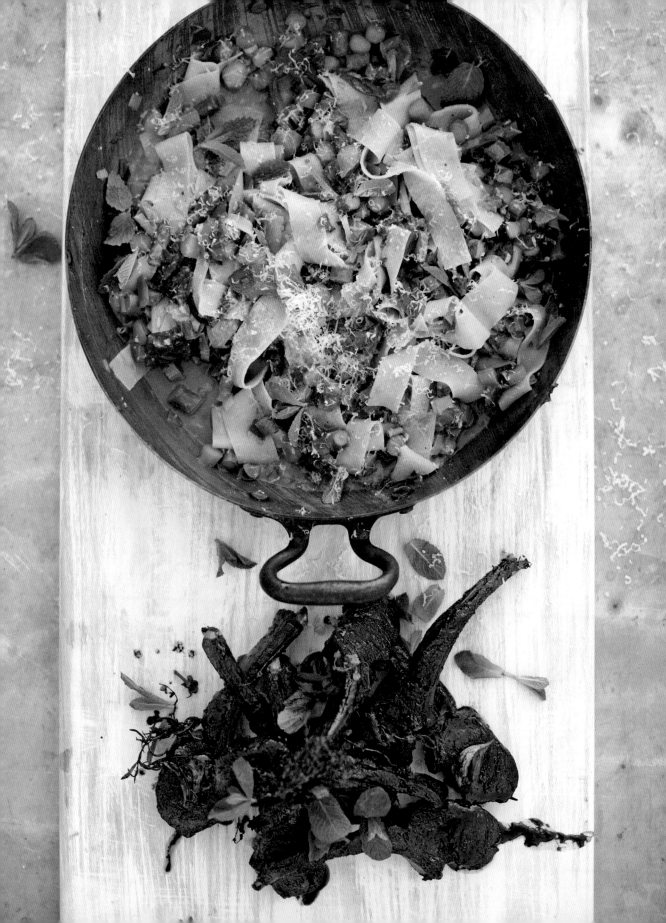

LAMB KOFTE
PITTA & GREEK SALAD

SERVES 4 | 587 CALORIES

Ingredients out • Kettle boiled • Large frying pan, high heat
• Food processor (bowl blade)

Kofte
400g lean lamb mince
1 tsp garam masala
olive oil
25g shelled pistachios
a few sprigs of fresh thyme
1 tbsp runny honey

Couscous
½ a bunch of fresh mint
1 fresh red chilli
½ a mug (150g) of couscous

Salad
½ an iceberg lettuce
½ a red onion
½ a cucumber
5 ripe cherry tomatoes
4 black olives (stone in)
4 heaped tbsp fat-free
    natural yoghurt
2 lemons
40g feta cheese

To serve
4 pitta breads

START COOKING

In a large bowl, mix the mince with salt, pepper and the garam masala • Divide into 8, then with wet hands shape into little fat fingers • Put into the frying pan with 1 tablespoon of oil, turning until dark golden all over • Tear off most of the top leafy half of the mint and blitz in the processor with a pinch of salt and pepper and the chilli until fine • Remove the blade, stir in ½ a mug of couscous and 1 mug of boiling water, put the lid on and leave to sit in the processor

Cut the lettuce into wedges and arrange on a nice board or platter • Peel and coarsely grate the onion and cucumber into a bowl, season well with salt, then squeeze out any excess salty liquid and sprinkle over the lettuce • Chop and add the tomatoes, then squash, destone and dot over the olives • Mix the yoghurt in a bowl with the juice of 1 lemon, season to taste, then drizzle it over the lettuce and crumble over the feta

Bash the pistachios in a pestle and mortar • Drain away the fat from the lamb, then toss with the bashed nuts, thyme leaves and honey, and turn the heat off • Pop the pittas in the microwave (800W) for 45 seconds to warm through, then cut in half and add to the board with the kofte • Fluff up the couscous, scatter the remaining mint leaves over everything and serve with lemon wedges

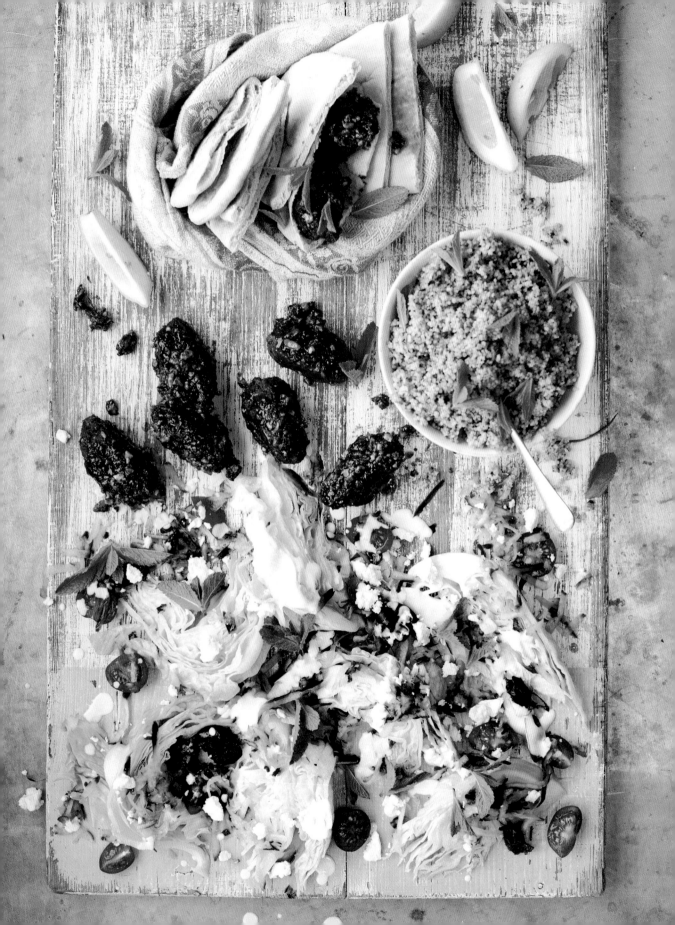

QUICK LAMB TAGINE
PAN-FRIED AUBERGINE & CUMIN CRUNCH

Ingredients out • Kettle boiled • Large frying pan, high heat
• Medium frying pan, medium heat

Lamb & aubergine
2 small aubergines
300g lamb neck fillet
1 heaped tsp garam masala
olive oil
a few sprigs of fresh coriander

Couscous
1 mug (300g) of couscous

Cumin crunch
1 heaped tbsp shelled pistachios
1 heaped tbsp sesame seeds
1 tbsp cumin seeds

Veg
1 good pinch of saffron
650g ripe mixed-colur tomatoes
1 preserved lemon
4 spring onions
½–1 fresh red chilli

To serve
4 tbsp fat-free natural yoghurt

START COOKING

Cook the aubergines whole in the microwave (800W) for 7 minutes • Put 1 mug of couscous and 2 mugs of boiling water into a bowl and cover • Cut the lamb into 8 pieces and flatten with your fist, then toss with salt, pepper and the garam masala • Put into the large frying pan with 1 tablespoon of oil, turning when golden • Toast the cumin crunch mix in the medium frying pan until lightly golden, then pound in a pestle and mortar • Return the empty pan to a low heat

Carefully transfer the aubergines to a board, then halve lengthways and add to the lamb pan, skin side down, pushing the lamb to the side • Put the saffron into a mug half-filled with boiling water • Roughly chop the tomatoes, finely chop the preserved lemon, trim and slice the spring onions and chilli, then add it all to the medium frying pan with 2 tablespoons of oil, the saffron and its soaking water • Turn the heat up to high, bring to the boil, then season to taste

Fluff up the couscous, then spoon over a large serving board or platter • Flip the aubergine over to soak up the pan juices, then place on top of the couscous and pour over the tomatoes and any juices • Lay over the lamb, then scatter with the cumin crunch and the coriander leaves • Serve with the yoghurt

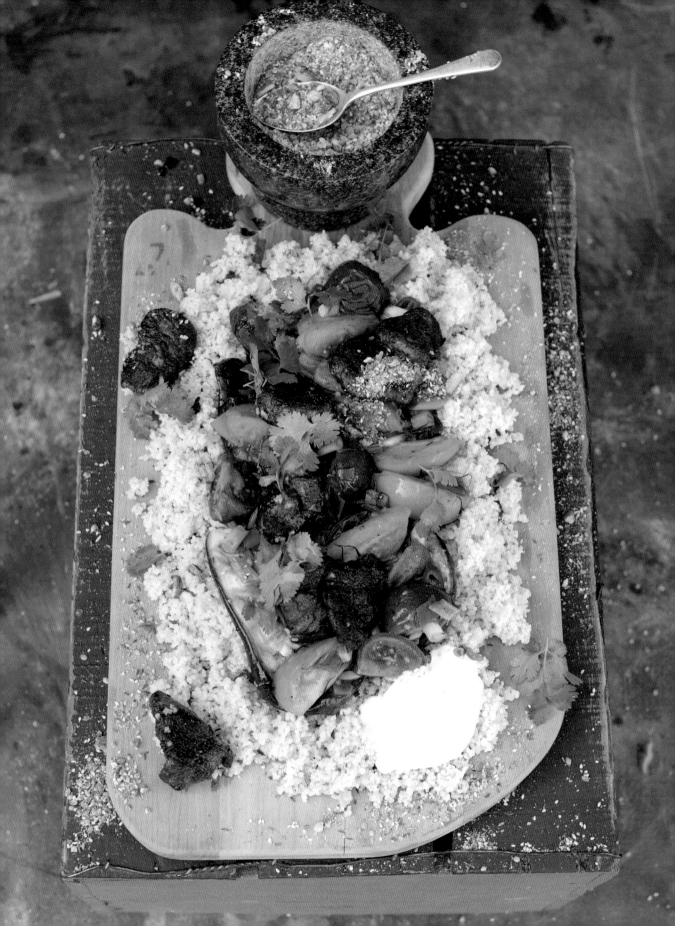

MUSTARD LAMB
IRISH MASH & WATERCRESS APPLE SALAD

SERVES 4 | 538 CALORIES

Ingredients out • Kettle boiled • Food processor (thick slicer & coarse grater)
• Medium lidded pan, high heat • Large frying pan, high heat

Mash

3 leeks
800g potatoes
semi-skimmed milk
1 whole nutmeg, for grating
optional: a knob of unsalted butter

Lamb

400g lamb neck fillet
2 tsp English mustard powder
rapeseed oil
1 heaped tbsp plain flour
250ml quality cider
2 heaped tsp mint sauce

Salad

1 inner celery heart
1 eating apple
100g watercress
1 bunch of fresh mint
1 tbsp cider vinegar

START COOKING

Split the leeks lengthways, rinse under the cold tap, then thickly slice with the potatoes in the processor, put into the medium pan with a pinch of salt, cover with boiling water and the lid and boil hard until tender, then drain – keep an eye on it • Score lengthways halfway through the centre of each piece of lamb and open out like a book • Sprinkle with salt, pepper and the mustard powder, then put into the frying pan with 1 tablespoon of oil, turning when golden

Swap to the coarse grater on your processor, pick and reserve any yellow celery leaves, then coarsely grate the stalks in the processor with the apple • Tip on to a platter with the watercress • Roughly chop and add the top leafy half of the mint • Drizzle with cider vinegar and 1 tablespoon of oil, season to taste and toss

Mash the drained potatoes and leeks, season well to taste, then loosen to your liking with a splash of milk, add a few scrapings of nutmeg and the butter, if using, and spoon on to a large platter • Transfer the lamb to a plate, then stir the flour into the lamb pan, followed by the cider • Pour in any lamb resting juices, then stir in the mint sauce and bring to the boil • Slice up the lamb and serve with the mash and gravy, scattered with the reserved celery leaves, and the salad on the side

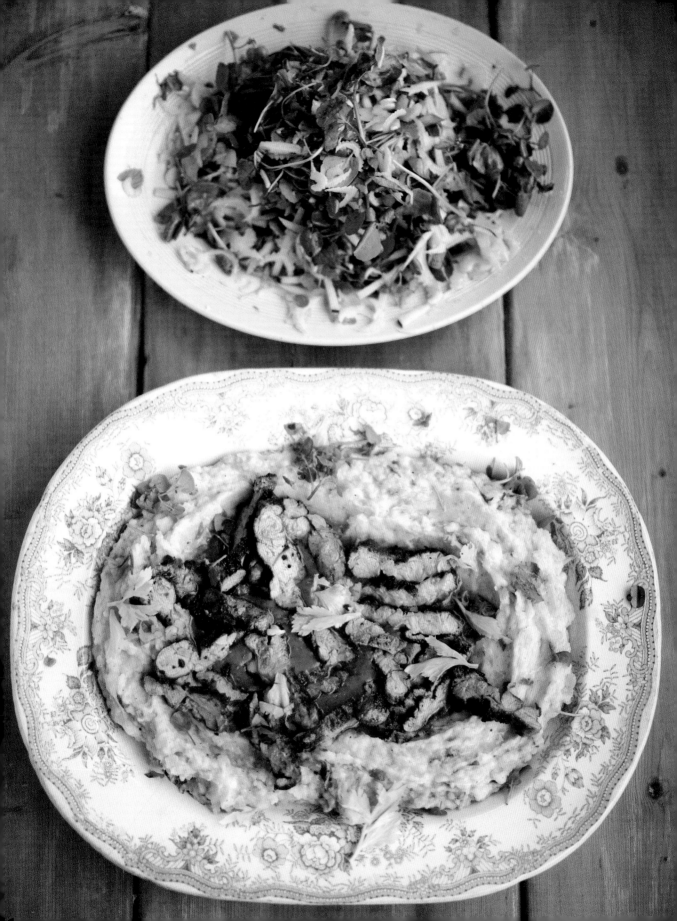

TURKISH FLATS
SHRED SALAD, FETA & HERBS

SERVES 4 | 525 CALORIES

Ingredients out • Oven at full whack (240°C/475°F/gas 9)
• Large frying pan, high heat • Food processor (fine slicer)

Flats
olive oil
250g lean lamb mince
1 tsp cumin seeds
1 tsp sweet smoked paprika
50g shelled walnuts
2 sprigs of fresh rosemary
2 cloves of garlic
2 tbsp tomato purée
1 lemon
4 large flour tortillas

Salad
4 spring onions
1 green pepper
¼ of a cucumber
3 ripe tomatoes
1 little gem lettuce
½ a bunch of fresh coriander
½ a bunch of fresh dill
1 tbsp extra virgin olive oil
1 tbsp red wine vinegar
30g feta cheese

To serve
4 heaped tsp low-fat houmous
optional: Lingham's chilli sauce
optional: pickled chillies

START COOKING

Put 1 tablespoon of olive oil into the frying pan with the mince, salt, pepper, cumin seeds and paprika • Crumble in the walnuts, strip in the rosemary leaves and break everything apart with a wooden spoon, stirring regularly until golden • Trim the spring onions, tear the stalks and seeds out of the pepper, then slice all the salad veg and herb leaves in the processor, tip on to a serving platter

Squash the unpeeled garlic through a garlic crusher into the lamb pan • Stir in the tomato purée and lemon juice, then take the pan off the heat • Lay the tortillas over 2 large baking trays and spread the lamb mixture evenly across them with the back of a spoon • Pop into the oven for 5 minutes to crisp up

Dress the salad veg with the extra virgin olive oil and vinegar, toss together then season to taste and crumble over the feta • Top and stuff the tortillas with loads of salad, then serve with houmous, and chilli sauce or pickled chillies, if you like

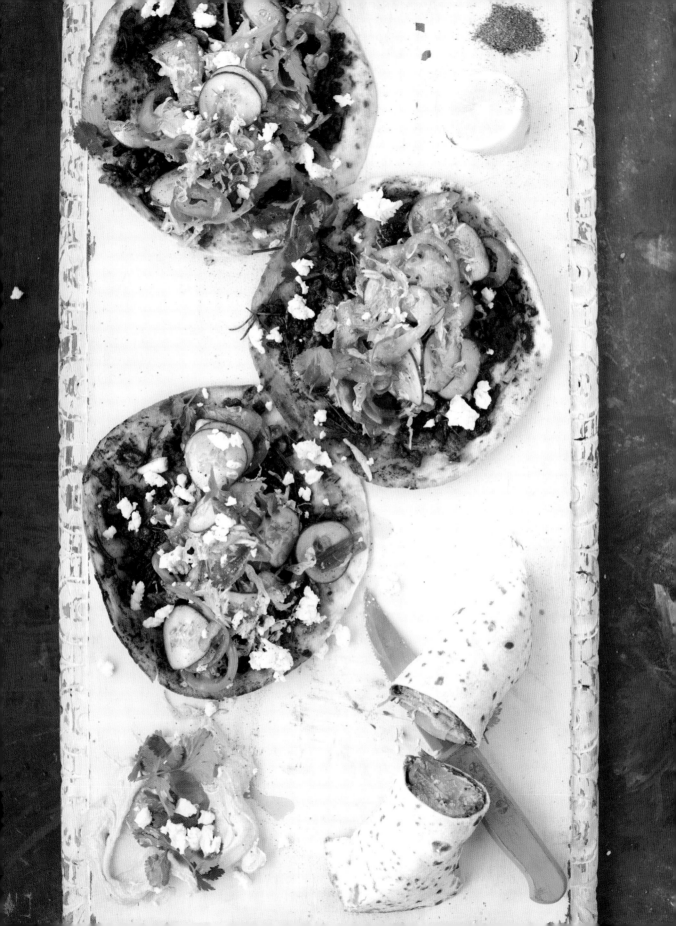

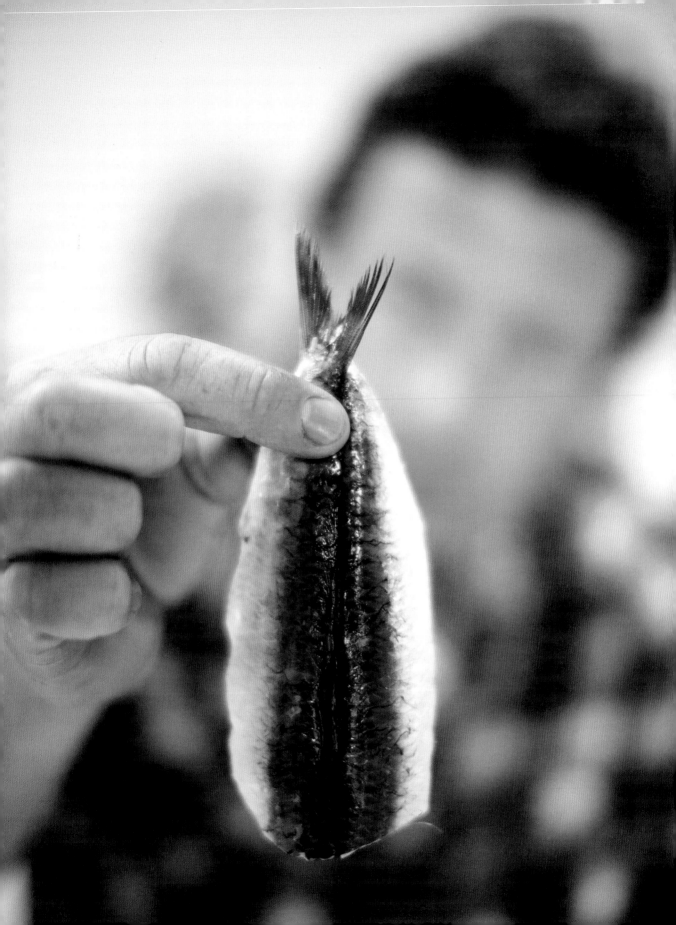

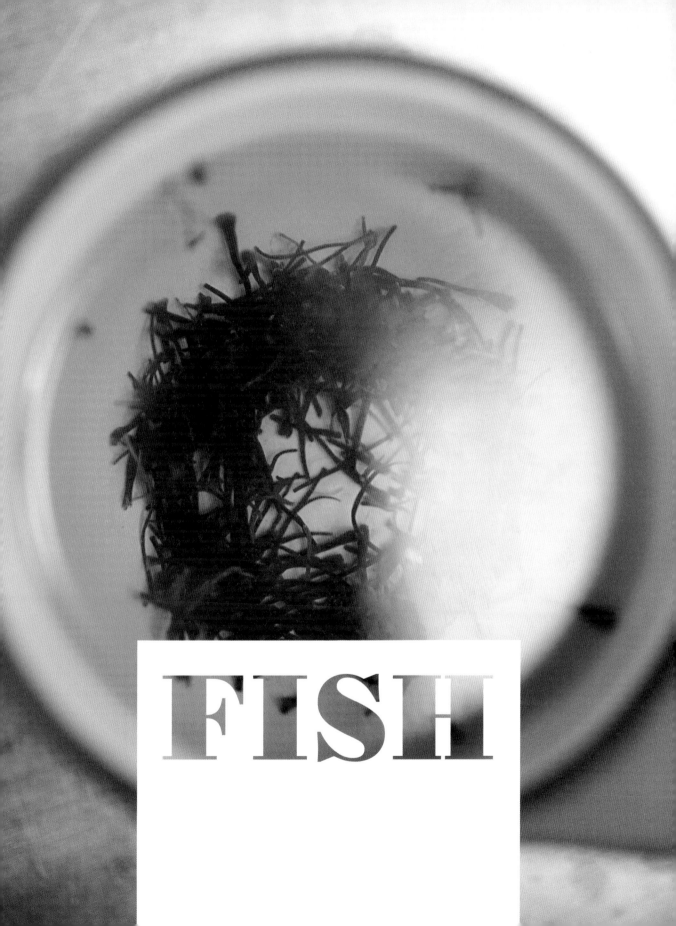

FISH

ASIAN SEA BASS
STICKY RICE & DRESSED GREENS

SERVES 4 | 629 CALORIES

Ingredients out • Kettle boiled • Medium lidded pan, medium heat • Casserole pan, medium heat • Food processor (bowl blade)

Fish

4 small whole sea bass or bream
(roughly 300g each), gutted and
scaled
1 thumb-sized piece of ginger
2 cloves of garlic
1 stick of lemongrass
1 bunch of fresh coriander
1 fresh red chilli
2 spring onions
3 tbsp low-salt soy sauce,
plus extra to serve
1 tbsp fish sauce
sesame oil
2 limes

Rice

1 x 400g tin of light coconut milk
1 coconut milk tin (300g)
of basmati rice

Greens

1 bunch of asparagus (300g)
2 bok choi
200g sugar snap peas
1 lime

START COOKING

Score the fish 5 times on each side down to the bone, then season all over and lay in a snug-fitting, high-sided tray • Pour in 400ml of boiling water, cover tightly with a double layer of tin foil and place on a medium-high heat to steam • Pour the coconut milk, 1 tin's worth of rice and 1 tin of boiling water (use a tea towel) into the medium pan • Add a pinch of salt, stir well, cover and cook for roughly 10 minutes, stirring ocasionally, then turn the heat off • Pour the rest of the boiling water into the casserole pan

Peel the ginger, garlic and the outer leaves of the lemongrass, roughly chop them and put into the processor • Add the coriander stalks (reserving the leaves), chilli, trimmed spring onions, soy and fish sauces, 1 teaspoon of oil and the juice of 2 limes to the processor and pulse until finely chopped, then pour into a bowl

Trim the asparagus, halve the bok choi and add both to the boiling water in the casserole pan with the sugar snaps • Cook for 2 minutes, then drain and toss with 1 tablespoon of oil and the juice of 1 lime, season to taste with soy sauce and serve with the fluffed-up rice • Uncover the fish, spoon some of its juices into the dressing, then pour everything back over the fish and serve scattered with coriander leaves

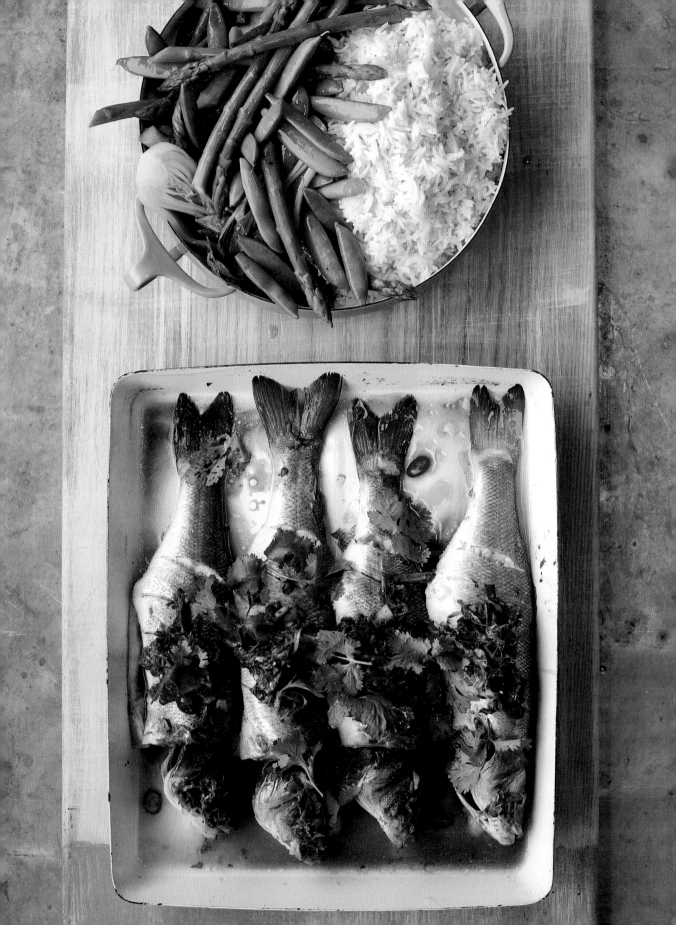

GRILLED CAJUN PRAWNS
SWEET POTATO MASH & HOLY TRINITY VEG

SERVES 4 | 396 CALORIES

Ingredients out • Kettle boiled • Oven grill on high • Food processor (thick slicer)
• Large lidded pan, high heat • Large frying pan, medium heat

Mash
800g sweet potatoes
40g Cheddar cheese

Prawns
16 large raw shell-on tiger prawns
3 cloves of garlic
1 heaped tbsp Cajun seasoning
olive oil
½ a bunch of fresh thyme
1 lemon

Veg
1 green pepper
1 red pepper
2 sticks of celery
5 spring onions
½ a fresh red chilli
1 big handful of frozen sweetcorn
1 tsp sweet smoked paprika

START COOKING

Wash the sweet potatoes and slice in the processor • Put into the lidded pan with a pinch of salt, then cover with boiling water and the lid • Put the prawns into a roasting tray, squash over the unpeeled garlic through a garlic crusher, then toss with the Cajun seasoning, 1 tablespoon of oil and the thyme sprigs • Spread out in a single layer and pop on a high heat for a couple of minutes to crisp the bottoms of the prawns up, then place under the grill until the tops are sizzling, golden and crispy

Deseed and roughly chop the peppers and put into the frying pan with 1 tablespoon of oil • Trim and slice the celery, spring onions and chilli, and add to the pan along with the sweetcorn and paprika • Season with salt and pepper and keep things moving

When cooked through, drain the sweet potatoes in a colander • Return to the pan and mash well • Grate in the cheese, mix well and season to taste • Scatter the veg over the mash and serve with the crispy prawns and lemon wedges

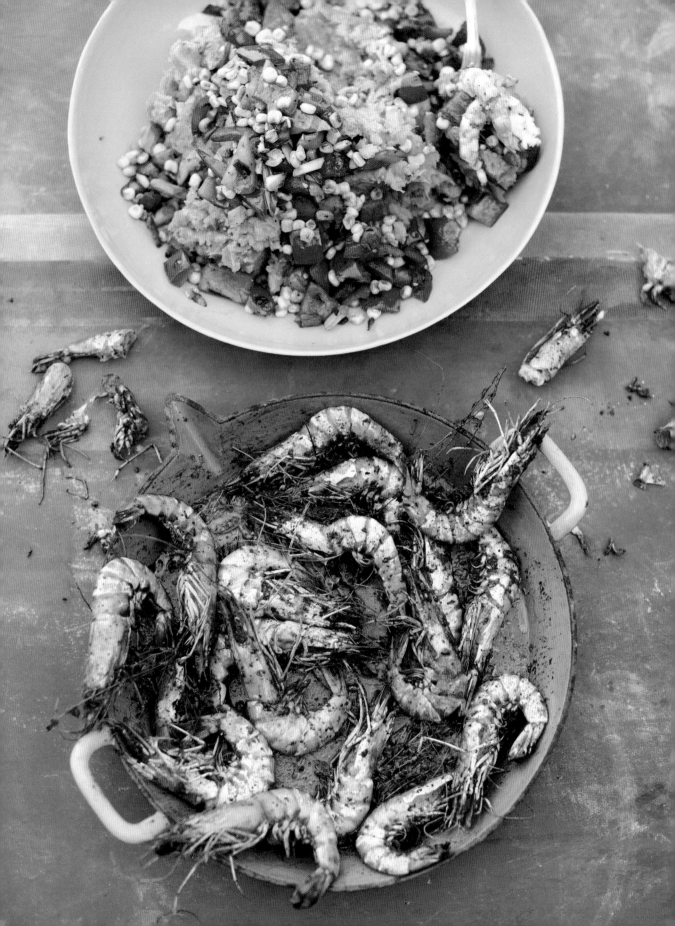

CRACKIN' CRAB BRIKS
COUSCOUS SALAD & SALSA

SERVES 4 | 457 CALORIES

Ingredients out • Kettle boiled • Large frying pan, medium heat • Food processor (coarse grater)

Briks

1–2 preserved lemons
2 spring onions
½ a bunch of fresh coriander
400g crabmeat (a mixture
    of brown and white meat)
2 tsp harissa, plus extra to serve
4 large sheets of filo pastry
    (from a 270g pack)
olive oil

Salad

½ tsp caraway seeds
½ a mug (150g) of couscous
2 tsp sun-dried tomato purée
½ a bulb of fennel
½ a bunch of fresh mint
1 lemon
extra virgin olive oil
1 pomegranate

Salsa

1 large ripe tomato
1 thumb-sized piece of ginger
½ a lemon

To serve

fat-free natural yoghurt

START COOKING

Finely chop the preserved lemons, trimmed spring onions and coriander (stalks and all) • Mix in a bowl with the crabmeat and harissa • Lay out a sheet of filo pastry, add ¼ of the mixture and shape into the size of a packet of playing cards at the centre of the bottom of the sheet, then push your thumb into the centre of the filling to make a space for it to expand as it cooks • Fold in the sides, then fold them up • Repeat until you have 4 briks • Put 1 tablespoon of olive oil into the pan, then add the briks and cook until golden and crisp on both sides • Add the caraway seeds to the side of the pan and toast for a minute, then scrape into a salad bowl

Put ½ a mug of couscous, 1 mug of boiling water, the tomato purée and a pinch of salt into a bowl and cover • Pick and reserve the fennel tops, then roughly chop and grate the bulb in the processor • Tip into the salad bowl, then chop and add the top leafy half of the mint • Squeeze in the lemon juice and drizzle with 1 tablespoon of extra virgin olive oil • Season to taste and toss everything together

Finely grate the tomato and ginger into a little bowl • Add a pinch of salt and pepper, a good squeeze of lemon juice and 1 tablespoon of extra virgin olive oil and mix together • Fluff up the couscous, then tip on to a platter • Pile the salad in the middle, then bash the halved pomegranate over the top so the seeds tumble out • Scatter over the reserved fennel tops, pop the crab briks on a board and serve with dollops of yoghurt and the salsa

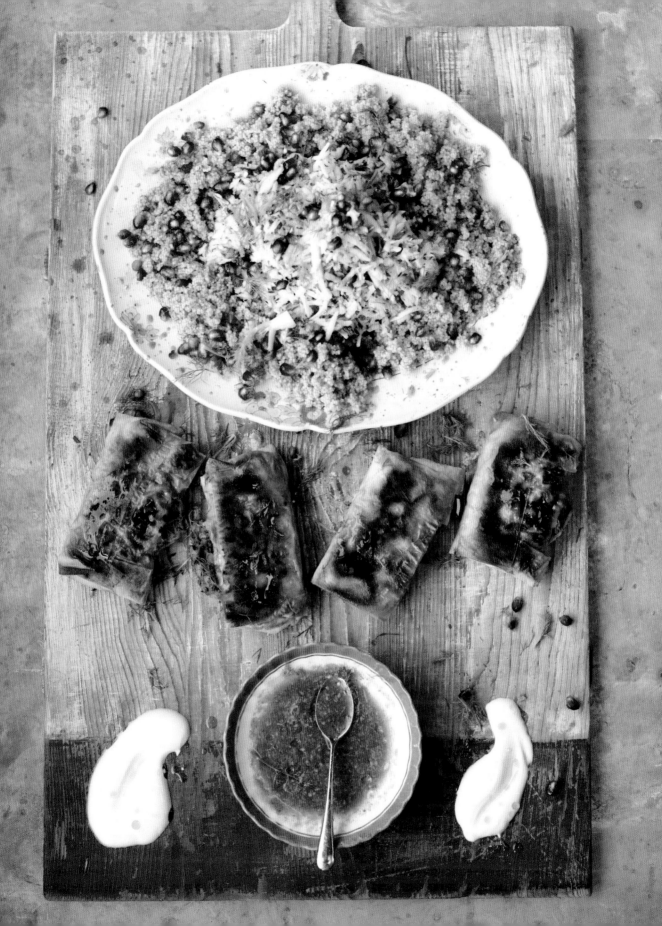

MIXED FISH GRILL
MEDITERRANEAN FENNEL & COUSCOUS

SERVES 4 | 458 CALORIES

Ingredients out • Kettle boiled • Oven at full whack (240°C/475°F/gas 9) • Large lidded pan, low heat • Food processor (fine slicer)

Fish

1 bunch of fresh flat-leaf parsley

1 fresh red chilli

12 ripe mixed-colour cherry
   tomatoes

2 cloves of garlic

olive oil

½ a lemon

400g mixed fish fillets (bream, sea
   bass, mullet or snapper), scaled
   and pin-boned

4 large raw shell-on king prawns

500g clams and mussels, scrubbed
   clean and debearded

Couscous

1 mug (300g) of couscous

Fennel

4 jarred sun-dried tomatoes

1 sprig of fresh rosemary

1 handful of mixed olives (stone in)

2 bulbs of fennel

1 lemon

To serve

1 lemon

4 tbsp fat-free natural yoghurt

START COOKING

Roughly chop the parsley leaves and chilli, and put into a large, high-sided roasting tray with the tomatoes • Squash in the unpeeled garlic through a garlic crusher and mix with 1 tablespoon of oil, salt, pepper and the juice of ½ a lemon • Halve the fish fillets, then add to the tray with the shellfish (throw away any mussels or clams that won't close when tapped), and toss together • Cook in the oven for 10 minutes, or until the clams and mussels have opened (throw away any that remain closed)

Put 1 mug of couscous, 2 mugs of boiling water and a pinch of salt and pepper into a bowl, then cover • Put the sun-dried tomatoes and a splash of their oil, the rosemary leaves and olives into the large pan • Halve the fennel bulbs, then finely slice in the processor, and add to the pan with a pinch of salt and the juice of 1 lemon • Turn the heat up to high and cover with the lid, stirring regularly

Fluff up the couscous • Season the fennel to taste • Serve with the tray of fish, lemon wedges and the yoghurt for dolloping over

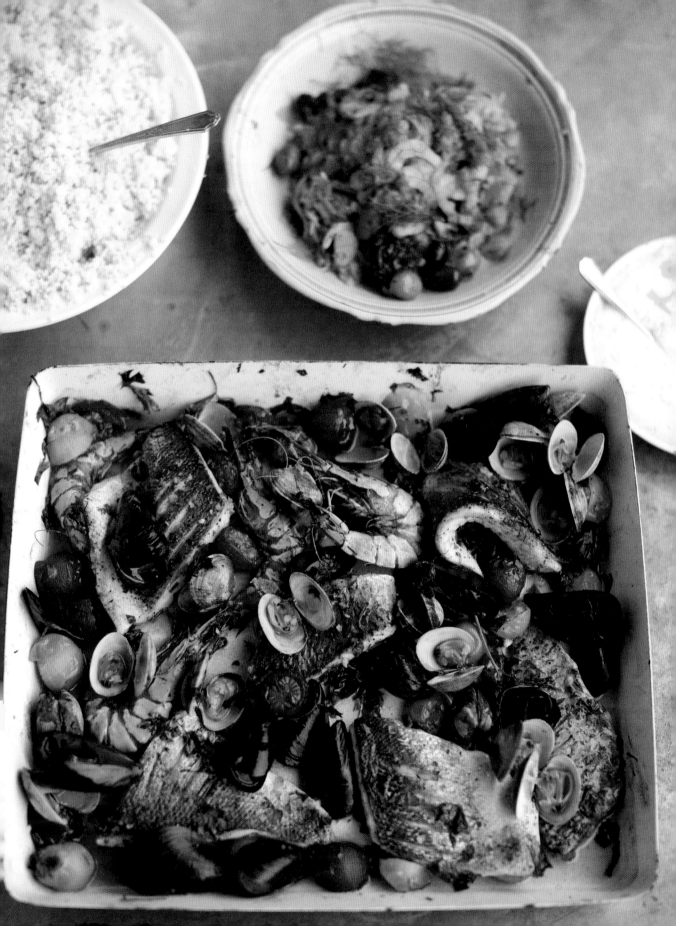

ASIAN FISH
MISO NOODLES & CRUNCHY VEG

SERVES 4 | 559 CALORIES

Ingredients out • Kettle boiled • Oven at 200°C/400°F/gas 6
• Casserole pan, high heat • Food processor (fine slicer)

Fish

2 tsp sesame oil

300g salmon fillet, skin off
  and pin-boned

300g of any white fish fillet,
  skin off and pin-boned

1 tbsp sesame seeds

1 lime

1 tbsp runny honey

2 sprigs of fresh coriander

Noodles

1 x 15g sachet of miso paste

2 tbsp low-salt soy sauce,
  plus extra to serve

5 dried kaffir lime leaves

3 nests of fine egg noodles

1 fresh red chilli

½ a cucumber

200g sugar snap peas

4 spring onions

1 little gem lettuce

200g radishes

1 lime

2 tbsp extra virgin olive oil

START COOKING

Rub half the sesame oil on a small shallow baking dish or ovenproof serving platter • Pat both fish dry with kitchen paper, slice them into 1cm-thick strips and arrange randomly around the dish or platter • Rub gently with the rest of the sesame oil and season with salt and pepper • Scatter over the sesame seeds, finely grate over the zest from 1 lime and squeeze over half the juice, then drizzle over the honey • Place in the oven to cook through (roughly 7 minutes)

Pour 1 litre of boiling water into the casserole pan with the miso paste, soy sauce, crumbled lime leaves and noodles, making sure they're fully submerged • Slice the chilli and add to the broth • Finely slice the cucumber, sugar snaps, trimmed spring onions, lettuce and radishes in the processor

Tip the sliced veg into a bowl and dress with the juice of 1 lime, a little soy sauce and the extra virgin olive oil • Check the noodles and switch off the heat when they're done, then season the broth to taste with soy sauce • Pile the veg in the centre of the noodles and toss together at the table • Serve the fish sprinkled with coriander leaves

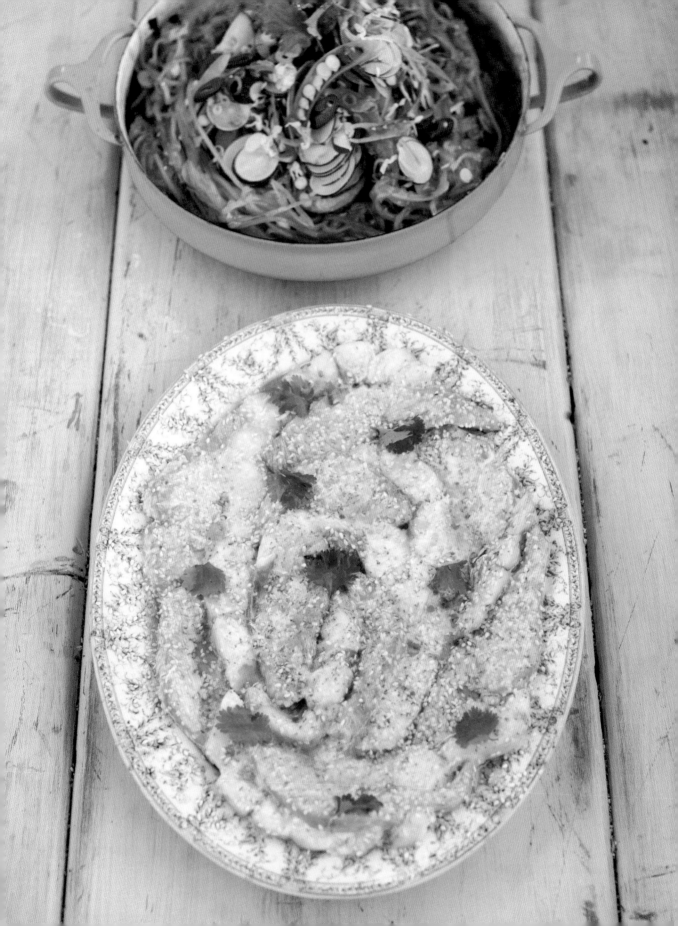

PRAWN COCKTAIL
KING PRAWNS & SUN-DRIED PAN BREAD

SERVES 4 | 525 CALORIES

Ingredients out • Food processor (bowl blade) • 28cm frying pan, medium heat • Medium frying pan, medium heat

Bread

200g self-raising flour, plus extra
  for dusting
100g jarred sun-dried tomatoes
3 sprigs of fresh basil
olive oil

Prawn cocktail

1 handful of mixed seeds
3 spring onions
1 romaine lettuce
½ a cucumber
3 ripe mixed-colour tomatoes
1 ripe avocado
1 punnet of cress
400g small cooked peeled prawns
4 heaped tbsp fat-free
  natural yoghurt
1 tsp Worcestershire sauce
1 tsp Tabasco
1 heaped tbsp tomato ketchup
1 tbsp brandy
1 lemon
1 tsp extra virgin olive oil

King prawns

1 good pinch of cayenne pepper
4 large raw shell-on king prawns
4 cloves of garlic

START COOKING

Blitz the flour, sun-dried tomatoes (drained) and basil in the processor, then gradually add small splashes of water to form a ball of dough • On a flour-dusted surface, shape the dough into a 28cm round • Put 1 tablespoon of olive oil and the dough into the 28cm pan, pat it out to the edges and cook until nicely golden, turning halfway (roughly 5 minutes on each side) • Put the seeds in the medium pan to toast, tossing often

Randomly slice up the trimmed spring onions, lettuce, cucumber and tomatoes on a nice serving board • Squeeze and squidge over the avocado flesh, discarding the skin and stone, and snip over the cress • Place the small prawns in the middle of the salad and pile the toasted seeds to one side, returning the pan to the heat • Add 1 tablespoon of olive oil to the medium pan with the cayenne pepper and king prawns, then squash in the unpeeled garlic through a garlic crusher, and fry, turning regularly until golden

In a bowl, mix the yoghurt with the Worcestershire sauce, Tabasco, ketchup, brandy and the juice from ½ a lemon, then season to taste • Spoon the sauce over the little prawns • When the king prawns are crispy, place on the board • Drizzle with a little extra virgin olive oil and lemon juice from a height and serve with torn-up pieces of the incredible pan bread

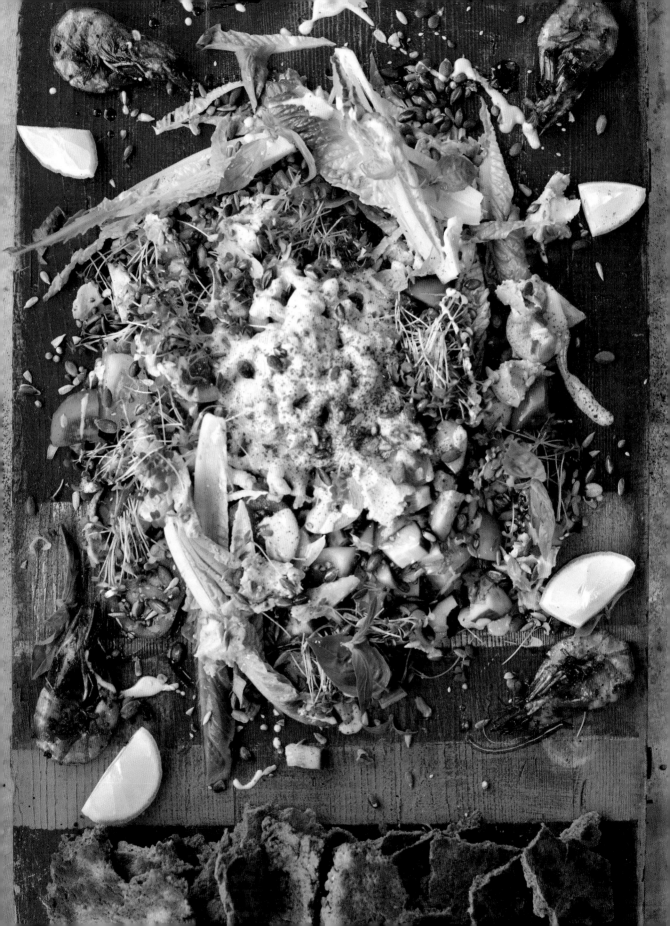

SMOKED SALMON
YORKSHIRE PUD, BEETS & ASPARAGUS

SERVES 4 | 407 CALORIES

Ingredients out • Oven at 200°C/400°F/gas 6
• 28cm non-stick ovenproof frying pan, high heat • Liquidizer
• Griddle pan, high heat • Casserole pan, medium heat

Yorkshire pud
olive oil
2 or 3 sprigs of fresh rosemary
2 large eggs
150ml semi-skimmed milk
65g plain flour
180g quality smoked salmon

Beets & asparagus
1 bunch of asparagus (300g)
250g vac-packed cooked beetroot
4 tbsp balsamic vinegar
1 heaped tsp runny honey
2 punnets of cress
2 sprigs of fresh basil
½ a lemon

Dressing
3 heaped tbsp fat-free natural
 yoghurt
2 heaped tbsp jarred
 grated horseradish
1 lemon

START COOKING

Put 2 tablespoons of oil into the frying pan and pick in the rosemary leaves • Crack the eggs into the liquidizer, add the milk and flour, then blitz until smooth • Spread out the rosemary in the pan, then pour in the batter, let it fry for 30 seconds, then pop into the oven and close the door until golden (roughly 13 minutes) • Trim the asparagus and put dry on the hot griddle pan, turning until nicely charred on all sides

Drain and slice or dice the beetroot, then place in the casserole pan with the balsamic and honey, stirring regularly, and removing from the heat when sticky • Mix the yoghurt and horseradish in a bowl, then season to taste with salt, pepper and lemon juice • Snip the cress on to a nice serving board, and spoon the beetroot on top, then pick over the basil leaves

Shake the asparagus with a squeeze of lemon juice, salt and pepper, and immediately pile on the board • Wait by the oven until your Yorkshire pudding is puffed up and beautiful • Once it looks so good you can't stand it any longer, get it out of the oven, slide it on to the board, then roll the smoked salmon into roses and place on top • Serve straight away with lemon wedges on the side

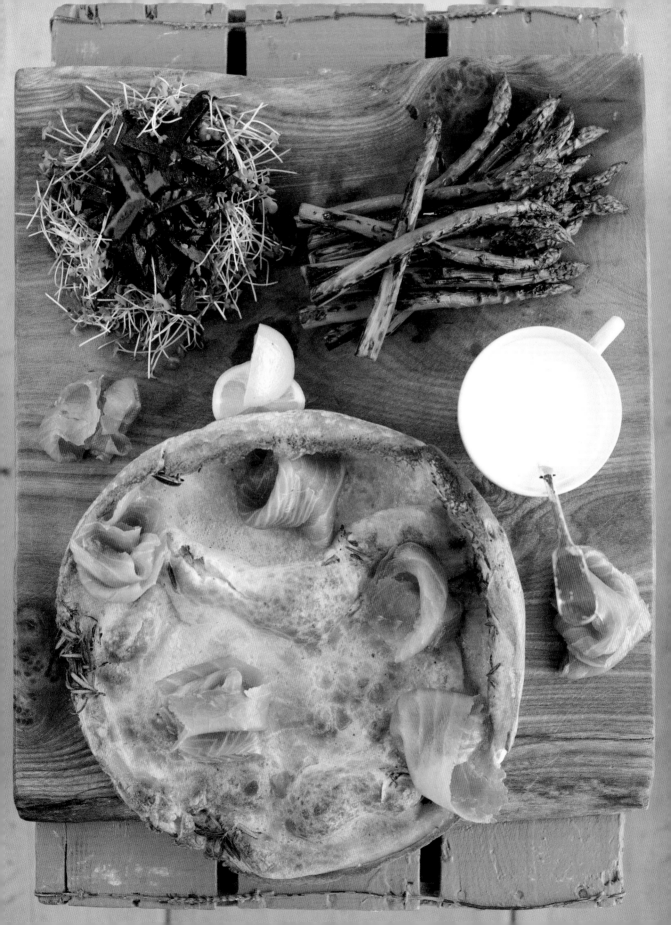

GRIDDLED TUNA
KINDA NIÇOISE SALAD

SERVES 4 | 491 CALORIES

Ingredients out • Kettle boiled • Medium lidded pan, high heat • Griddle pan, high heat • Liquidizer

Salad

350g mixed green and
   yellow beans
½ a baguette
12 black olives (stone in)
3 ripe mixed-colour tomatoes
1 romaine lettuce
20g feta cheese
1 lemon

Tuna & dressings

1 big bunch of fresh basil
6 anchovy fillets
1 lemon
4 tbsp extra virgin olive oil
2 x 200g tuna steaks (2.5cm thick)
1 tbsp red wine vinegar
1 heaped tsp wholegrain mustard
1 tsp runny honey

START COOKING

Line the beans up and cut off the stalks, put them into the pan with a pinch of salt, then cover with boiling water and the lid • Slice the baguette into 2cm chunks and put on the griddle pan, turning when golden • Pick and reserve 10 baby sprigs of basil • Rip off the rest of the leaves and blitz them in the liquidizer with the anchovies, juice of 1 lemon, the extra virgin olive oil and a splash of water

Pour about 40% of the dressing on to a nice serving platter and put aside • Rub 10% into the tuna and season with salt and pepper • Pour the rest of the dressing into a big bowl with the vinegar, mustard and honey, then mix together • Drain the cooked beans, remove the stones from the olives, roughly chop the tomatoes, then add it all to the bowl of dressing and toss together

Put the tuna on the griddle pan and cook for 2 minutes on each side, or until blushing in the middle • Chop the lettuce into 2cm chunks, tear the toasts into croutons and arrange over a large board with the lettuce • Scatter the dressed beans, olives and tomatoes over the top • Tear each tuna steak in half and add to the dressing platter • Scatter over the reserved basil leaves, crumble over the feta and serve with lemon wedges

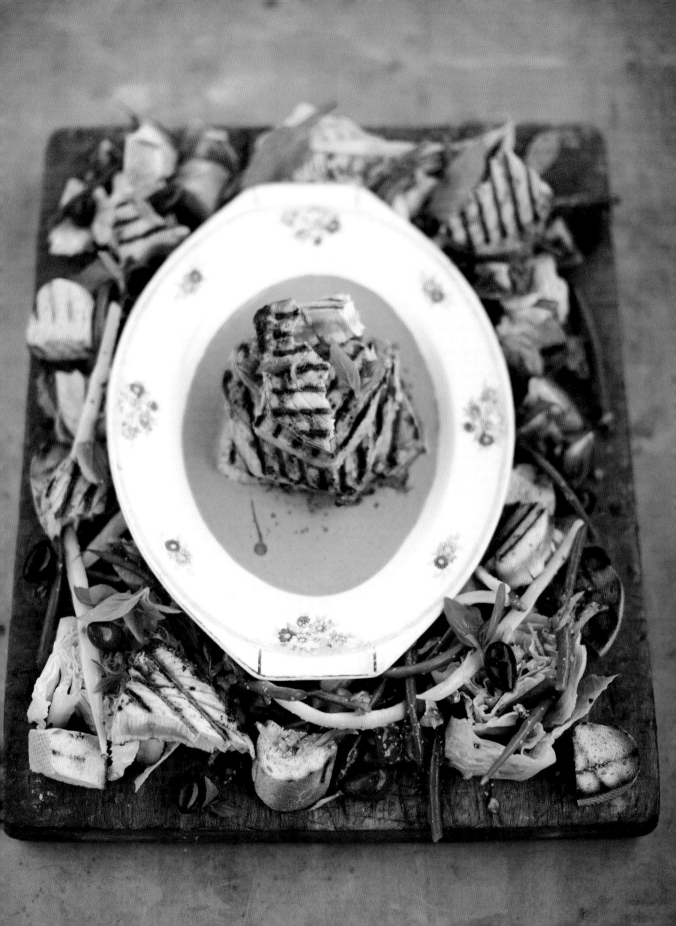

STICKY SQUID BALLS
GRILLED PRAWNS & NOODLE BROTH

SERVES 4 | 489 CALORIES

Ingredients out • Kettle boiled • Large lidded pan, high heat
• Food processor (fine slicer & bowl blade) • Large frying pan, medium heat

Broth

2 chicken stock cubes

400g sugar snap peas

½ a Chinese white cabbage

2 fresh red chillies

200g tenderstem broccoli

2 bok choi

1 bunch of radishes

1 thumb-sized piece of ginger

1 tbsp fish sauce

2 tbsp low-salt soy sauce

4 nests of egg noodles

2 limes

Squid & prawns

225g fresh squid, gutted
   and cleaned

½ a bunch of fresh coriander

1 tbsp sesame oil

225g large raw peeled tiger prawns

sweet chilli sauce

1 tbsp sesame seeds

START COOKING

Pour 1.5 litres of boiling water into the large pan and crumble in the stock cubes • Slice the sugar snaps, cabbage and 1 chilli in the processor, then tip into a large bowl • Trim the ends off the broccoli, quarter the bok choi and add both to the bowl, along with the radishes • Finely grate half the peeled ginger and finely slice half a chilli, then add both to the stock with the fish and soy sauces, and cover with a lid

Swap to the bowl blade, add the remaining chilli and ginger, the squid (pat dry with kitchen paper first), coriander stalks, salt and pepper, then blitz to a paste, using a spatula to scrape the mixture from the sides after a minute • Put the sesame oil into the frying pan • Use 2 dessert spoons to scrape and dollop the squid around the pan so you get 8 balls • Fry, turning when nicely golden, and adding the prawns after turning

Stir the noodles and veg into the stock, pop the lid back on and bring back to the boil • Turn the prawns, drizzle over some sweet chilli sauce, scatter over the sesame seeds, then gently shake the pan to coat • Squeeze the limes into the broth, stir and season to perfection • Ladle the noodles, veg and broth into bowls and serve the seafood on top • Finish with the coriander leaves

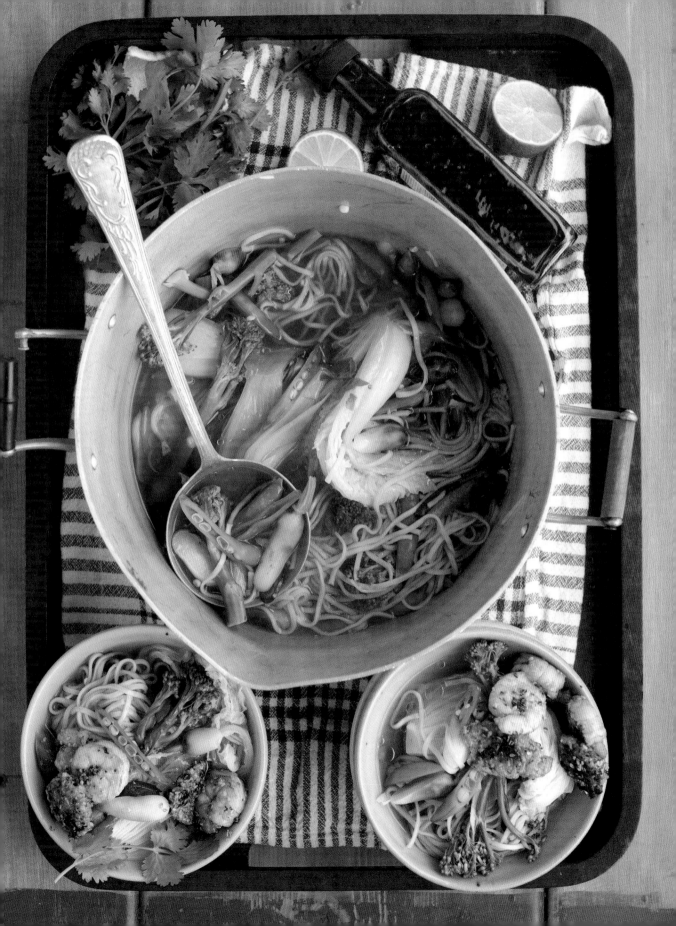

MOROCCAN BREAM
COUSCOUS, POMEGRANATE & HARISSA

SERVES 4 | 611 CALORIES

Ingredients out • Kettle boiled • Large frying pan, medium-high heat
• Food processor (bowl blade)

Fish

4 x 300g whole bream, heads
and tails removed, scaled
and gutted
olive oil
1 big pinch of saffron
4 spring onions
a few sprigs of fresh thyme
1 tsp harissa, plus extra to serve

Couscous & salsa

1 mug (300g) of couscous
1 preserved lemon
70g dried apricots
6 jarred red peppers
1 bunch of fresh coriander
1 pomegranate

To serve

2 tbsp shelled pistachios
1 tbsp sesame seeds
4 heaped tbsp fat-free natural
yoghurt
1 tsp rosewater

START COOKING

Toast the pistachios and sesame seeds in the pan for 1 minute, then remove and place the pan back on the heat • Score the fish in a crisscross fashion on both sides down to the bone • Season all over with salt and pepper and add to the pan with 1 tablespoon of oil, then cook for 3 minutes on each side • Put 1 mug of couscous, 2 mugs of boiling water and a pinch of salt into a bowl and cover • Cover the saffron with 150ml boiling water

Blitz the preserved lemon, apricots, peppers and half the coriander in the processor until fine, then spoon into a bowl, squeeze in the juice of ½ the pomegranate, mix, season to taste and put aside • Slice the trimmed spring onions and add to the fish with the thyme sprigs, harissa, saffron and soaking water • Scrunch up and wet a sheet of greaseproof paper and tuck it over the fish

Spoon the yoghurt into a small bowl, then marble through the rose water and a little harissa • Fluff up the couscous, tip it over a warm platter or board and spoon over the salsa • Lay the fish on top, spoon over some of the juices, then scatter over the toasted nuts and seeds • Hold the second pomegranate half in the palm of your hand and bash the back of it with a spoon so the seeds tumble over the salad • Finish with the rest of the coriander leaves

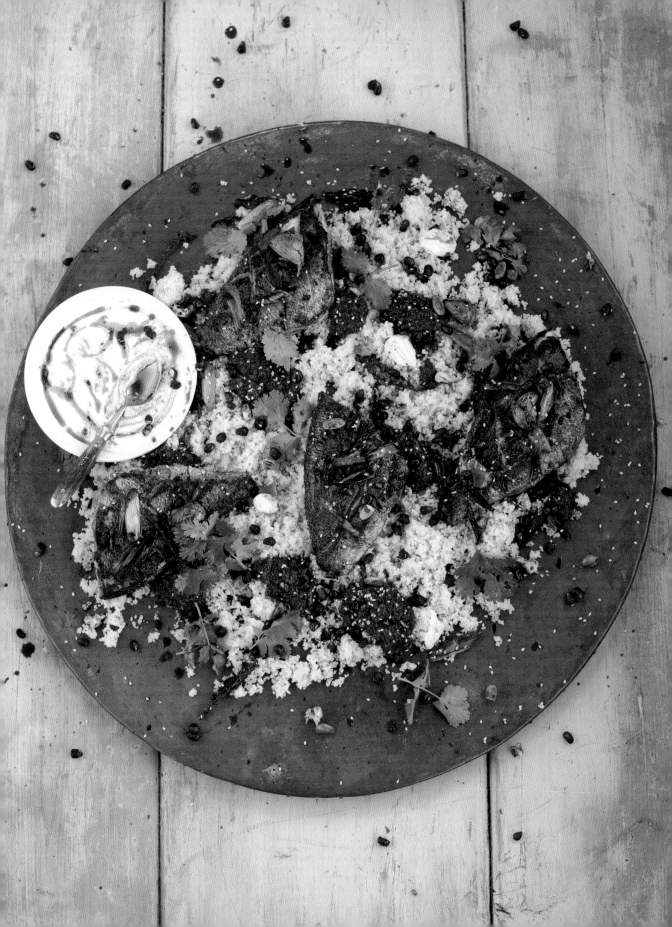

GREEN TEA SALMON
COCONUT RICE & MISO GREENS

SERVES 4 | 603 CALORIES

Ingredients out • Kettle boiled • Large frying pan, medium-high heat • Large lidded pan, medium heat • Medium lidded pan, medium heat • Liquidizer

Salmon
4 x 120g salmon fillets, skin on,
  scaled and pin-boned
2 green tea bags
olive oil

Rice
1 x 400g tin of light coconut milk
1 coconut milk tin (300g)
  of basmati rice
½ a lemon

Greens
½–1 fresh red chilli
1 small thumb-sized piece of ginger
1 heaped tsp miso powder
  or 1 tbsp miso paste
½ a bunch of fresh coriander
½ a lemon
2–3 tbsp low-salt soy sauce
1 heaped tsp runny honey
200g sugar snap peas
200g tenderstem broccoli
1 bunch of asparagus (300g)
1 lime

START COOKING

Put the salmon on a plate, rip open the green tea bags and scatter the contents over the fish, season with salt and pepper and rub in • Put into the frying pan, skin side down, with 1 teaspoon of oil, turning until golden on all sides • Pour the coconut milk, 1 tin's worth of rice and 1 tin of boiling water (use a tea towel) into the large pan • Add ½ a lemon, stir well, cover and cook for roughly 10 minutes, stirring occasionally, then turn the heat off

Finely slice ½ the chilli for garnish and throw the rest into the liquidizer with the peeled ginger, the miso powder or paste, most of the coriander, the juice of ½ a lemon, the soy sauce, honey and a splash of water, then whiz until smooth • Pour the rest of the kettle water into the medium pan • Add the sugar snaps, trimmed broccoli and asparagus and a pinch of salt and cook for a few minutes, until just tender

Remove the cooked salmon from the pan, gently pull the skins off and put back soft-side down to crisp up for 30 seconds • Pour the dressing on to a platter, then quickly drain the greens and place nicely on top • Fluff up the rice, then flake the salmon over the top, sprinkle with the chilli and the rest of the coriander leaves, then serve with the crispy salmon skin and lime wedges

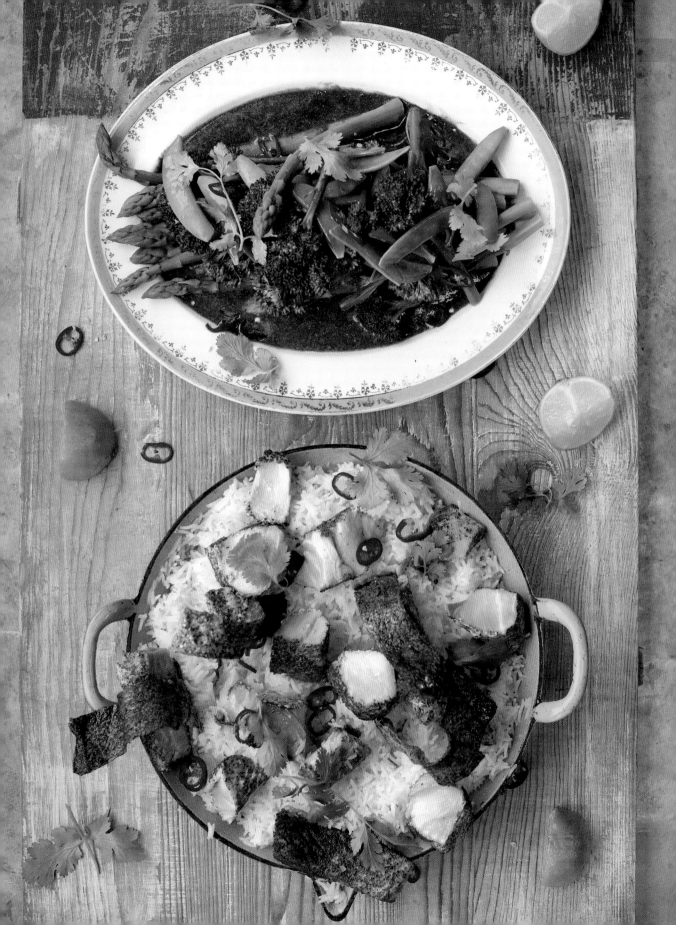

ARNOLD BENNETT FRITTATA
FOCACCIA & EMMENTAL WALDORF SALAD

SERVES 4 | 569 CALORIES

Ingredients out • Kettle boiled • Oven grill on high • Large casserole pan, high heat • 26cm non-stick ovenproof frying pan, medium heat

Frittata
250g undyed smoked haddock
4 fresh bay leaves
8 large eggs
6 spring onions
½ a bunch of fresh mint
1 large handful of frozen peas
olive oil
5g Parmesan cheese

Salad
2 apples
1 lemon
½ a bunch of fresh chives
1 handful of walnuts
75g watercress
2 tbsp extra virgin olive oil
30g Emmental cheese

To serve
200g focaccia bread
1 lemon

START COOKING

Put the fish and bay leaves into the casserole pan and cover with boiling water • Pop the focaccia on the very bottom shelf of the grill to toast • Beat the eggs in a large bowl with a pinch of salt and pepper • Trim and finely slice the spring onions and the top leafy part of the mint and mix into the eggs, along with the peas

Use a fish slice to remove the fish to a bowl, then flake with a fork, discarding the skin • Turn the heat under the frying pan up to high, add 1 tablespoon of olive oil and pour in the egg mixture • Stir for a minute until it begins to set • Sprinkle over the poached haddock, finely grate over a dusting of Parmesan then put the pan under the grill on the top shelf until cooked through, fluffy and golden (roughly 5 minutes)

On a nice large board, matchstick or coarsely grate the apples, then quickly squeeze over some lemon juice to stop them discolouring • Finely chop the chives and sprinkle them over the apple • Crumble over the walnuts, add the watercress and drizzle with the extra virgin olive oil, then toss together and season to taste • Speed-peel slices of Emmental over the top • Get the frittata and focaccia out from under the grill and serve straight away with lemon wedges

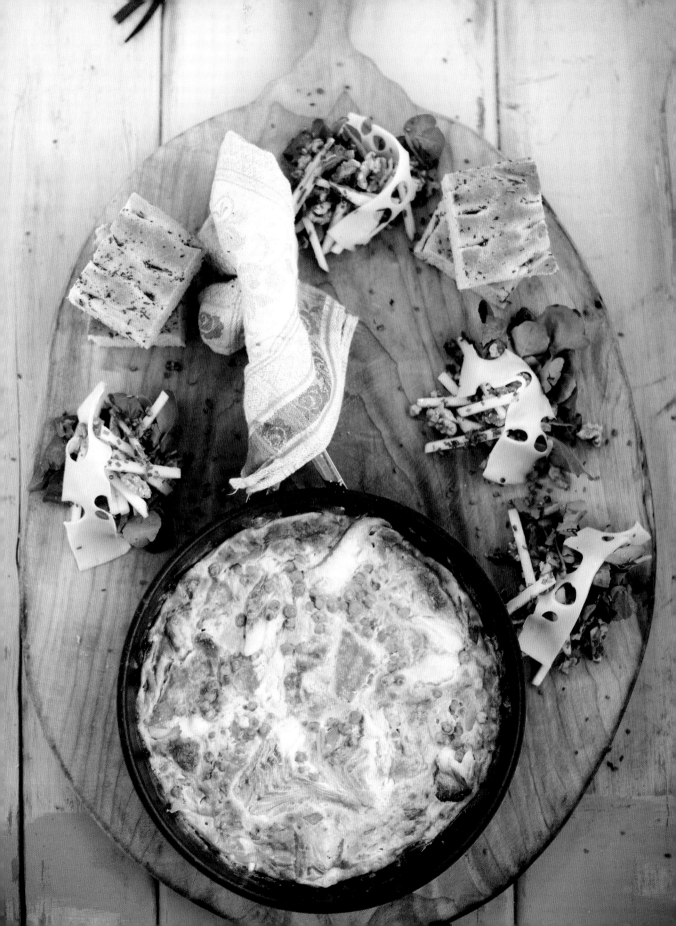

MOROCCAN MUSSELS
TAPENADE TOASTIES & CUCUMBER SALAD

SERVES 4 | 549 CALORIES

Ingredients out • *Large high-sided roasting tray, low heat* • *Liquidizer* • *Large griddle pan, high heat*

Mussels
olive oil
3 cloves of garlic
2 heaped tsp harissa
2 x 400g tins of chopped tomatoes
½ a bunch of fresh coriander
2 preserved lemons
1 pinch of saffron
2½kg mussels, scrubbed clean
    and debearded

To serve
1 ciabatta loaf
1 small soft round lettuce
½ a cucumber
a few sprigs of fresh mint
½ a lemon
4 tbsp fat-free natural yoghurt
½ a clove of garlic
90g jar of sun-dried tomato
    tapenade

START COOKING

Pour 2 tablespoons of oil into the roasting tray • Squash in the unpeeled garlic through a garlic crusher and stir in the harissa • Pour the tomatoes into the liquidizer with most of the coriander, salt, pepper, the preserved lemons and the saffron, purée, then pour into the tray and turn the heat up

Bring the sauce to the boil, then stir in the mussels (throw away any open ones that don't close when tapped) and cover well with a double layer of tin foil, pinching it at the sides to seal (use a tea towel to protect your hands) • Cut the ciabatta lengthways into quarters and put on the griddle pan, turning when golden and charred • Cut the lettuce into quarters and place on a big board

Using a box grater, coarsely grate the cucumber in long strokes, add a good pinch of salt, then toss and squeeze to get rid of the excess salty liquid, and pop in a bowl • Rip off the top leafy half of the mint, finely chop it and add to the cucumber with the lemon juice and yoghurt, then season to taste and spoon over the lettuce • Rub the toast with ½ a garlic clove and spread over the tapenade • Check to see if the mussels have opened up (throw away any that remain closed), then sprinkle with the remaining coriander leaves, correct the seasoning of the sauce and serve with the toasties and salad

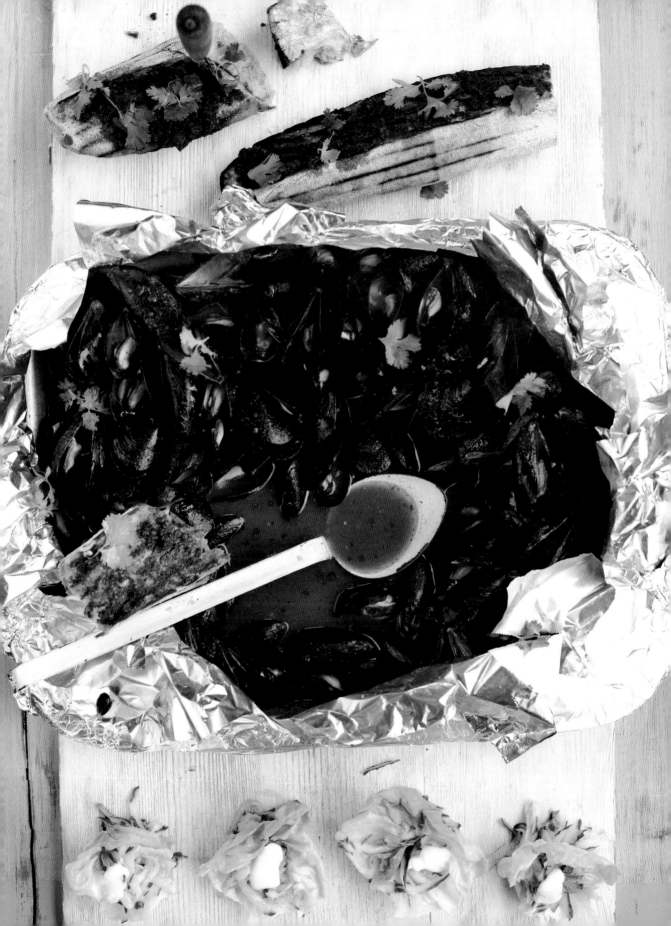

GOLDEN SCALLOPS
SUN-BLUSH MASH & GREENS

SERVES 4 | 441 CALORIES

Sun-blush mash
800g potatoes
40g Cheddar cheese
70g jarred sun-dried
   tomatoes in oil
optional: 1 splash of milk

Veg
200g tenderstem broccoli
200g asparagus spears
200g frozen peas
1 tbsp extra virgin olive oil
½ a lemon

Scallops
4 rashers of smoked
   streaky bacon
12 large scallops
olive oil
20 fresh sage leaves
½ a lemon

Ingredients out • Kettle boiled • Large shallow lidded casserole pan, high heat
• Medium pan, high heat • Food processor (bowl blade)
• Large frying pan, medium heat

START COOKING

Slice the potatoes 1cm thick, put into the casserole pan with a pinch of salt, then cover with boiling water and the lid • Refill and boil the kettle • Trim the ends off the broccoli and asparagus (I like to put the asparagus through a runner bean cutter, if you've got one, or you can leave them whole) • Put both veg into the medium pan with the peas, cover with boiling water and cook for 3 minutes • Drain, toss with the extra virgin olive oil and the juice of ½ a lemon, and put into a serving bowl

Crumble the cheese into the processor, add the sun-dried tomatoes and ½ a tablespoon of their oil and blitz well • Finely slice the bacon • Pat the scallops dry with kitchen paper, then score on one side in deep crisscrosses and season with salt and pepper • Put 1 tablespoon of olive oil into the hot frying pan and add the scallops, scored side down • Cook until lightly golden on both sides, then add the bacon and sage leaves

Drain the potatoes, tip into the processor and pulse up (oozy is good, but over-blitz and the mash will go gluey – not good), loosen with a splash of milk if needed • Check the seasoning and spoon on to a serving platter • Squeeze the juice of ½ a lemon over the scallops, shake and toss the pan, then serve right away with the veg on the side

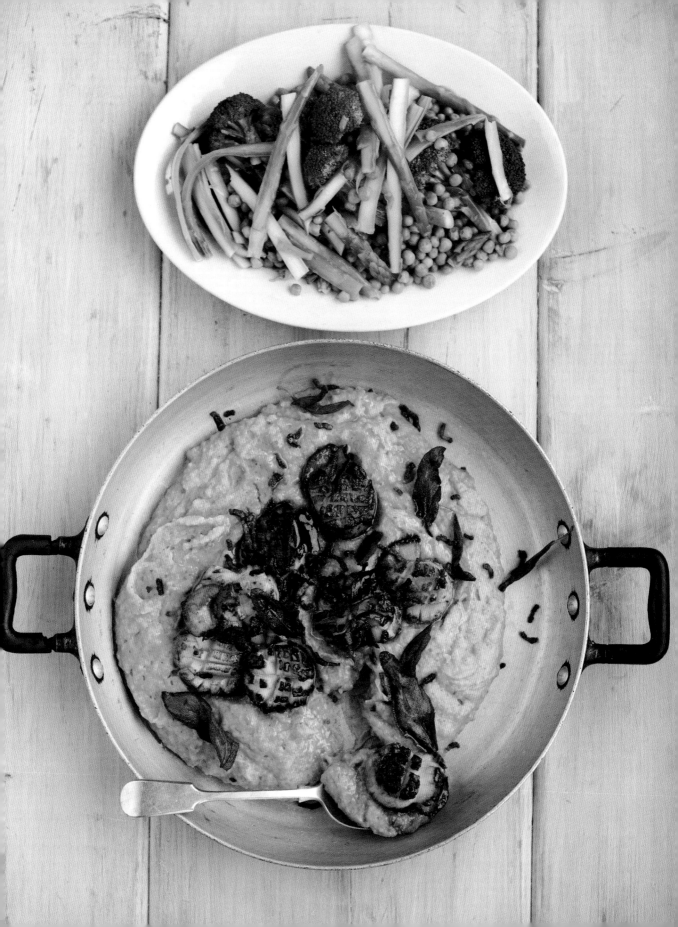

KILLER KEDGEREE
BEANS, GREENS & CHILLI YOGHURT

SERVES 4 | 474 CALORIES

Ingredients out • Kettle boiled • Large frying pan, high heat
• Large casserole pan, medium heat • Medium lidded pan, medium heat

Kedgeree

2 large eggs
4 fresh bay leaves
450g of any undyed smoked
    white fish fillets, scaled and
    pin-boned
1 thumb-sized piece of ginger
1 fresh red chilli
1 bunch of spring onions
1 bunch of fresh coriander
2 heaped tsp mustard seeds
2 heaped tsp turmeric
olive oil
2x 250g packs of brown
    cooked rice
300g frozen peas
1 lemon

Greens

200g fine green beans
1 big bunch of chard
1 tbsp extra virgin olive oil
½ a lemon

Yoghurt

3 tbsp fat-free natural yoghurt
1 tbsp sweet chilli sauce
½ a lemon

START COOKING

Fill the frying pan with boiling water, add the eggs, bay leaves and smoked fish, then reduce to a simmer • Refill and boil the kettle • Finely chop or slice the peeled ginger, chilli, trimmed spring onions and coriander (reserving a few leaves) • Put the mustard seeds and turmeric into the casserole pan with 1 tablespoon of olive oil, and when they pop, scrape in the chopped veg from the board, stirring regularly

Line the beans up and cut off the stalks, put into the medium pan with a pinch of salt, then cover with boiling water and the lid • Line up your chard leaves, cut off and slice the stalks and add the stalks to the beans • Stir the cooked rice, peas and the juice from 1 lemon into the casserole pan • Add the chard leaves to the beans for a minute • Ripple the yoghurt, chilli sauce and the juice of ½ a lemon together in a bowl

Drain the greens and leave to steam dry • Use a fish slice to remove the smoked fish from the pan, flake it into the rice, discarding the skin, stir and mix up beautifully, then season to taste • Peel the eggs under the cold tap and cut into quarters, place around the kedgeree pan and scatter over the reserved coriander leaves • Dress the greens on a board with the extra virgin olive oil and lemon juice, then season to taste and serve

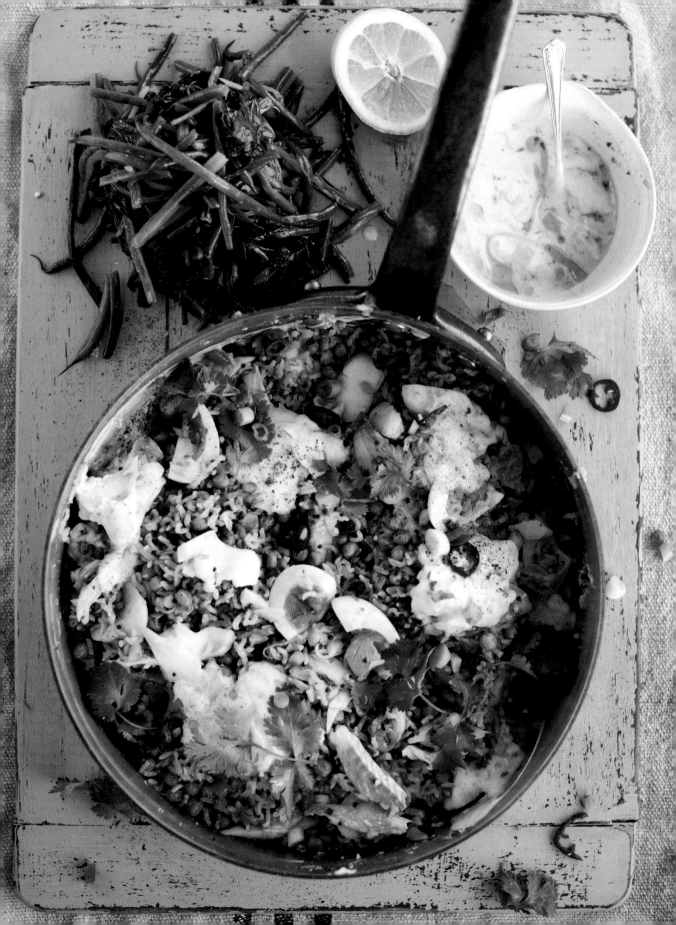

MIGHTY MACKEREL
MIXED TOMATO & QUINOA SALAD

SERVES 4 | 431 CALORIES

Ingredients out • Kettle boiled • Medium lidded pan, medium heat
• Large frying pan, high heat

Salad
1 mug (300g) of quinoa
½ a lemon
800g ripe mixed-colour tomatoes
1 fresh red chilli
2 tbsp extra virgin olive oil
1 tbsp balsamic vinegar

Mackerel
4 x 200g whole mackerel,
  scaled and gutted
1 heaped tsp ground coriander
olive oil
2 sprigs of fresh rosemary
2 cloves of garlic

To serve
2 heaped tbsp fat-free natural
  yoghurt
2 heaped tsp jarred grated
  horseradish
a couple of sprigs of fresh basil

START COOKING

Put 1 mug of quinoa and 2 mugs of boiling water into the medium pan with a pinch of salt and the lemon half, then pop the lid on and stir every now and again • On greaseproof paper, score the mackerel on both sides at 2cm intervals down to the bone • Rub all over with salt, pepper and the ground coriander, then put into the large frying pan with 1 tablespoon of olive oil

Slice the tomatoes any way you like and arrange on a large board or platter, then finely slice and sprinkle over the chilli • Strip the rosemary leaves over the fish, then crush and add the whole garlic cloves • Turn the fish when golden (roughly 4 to 5 minutes on each side)

When the quinoa is cooked (after roughly 10 minutes), drain it and use tongs to squeeze over the lemon juice, then spoon the quinoa into the centre of the tomatoes • Drizzle with the extra virgin olive oil and balsamic, and a pinch of salt and pepper • Lay the crispy fish on top • Mix the yoghurt and horseradish together and dollop it over the fish • Pick over the basil leaves and serve

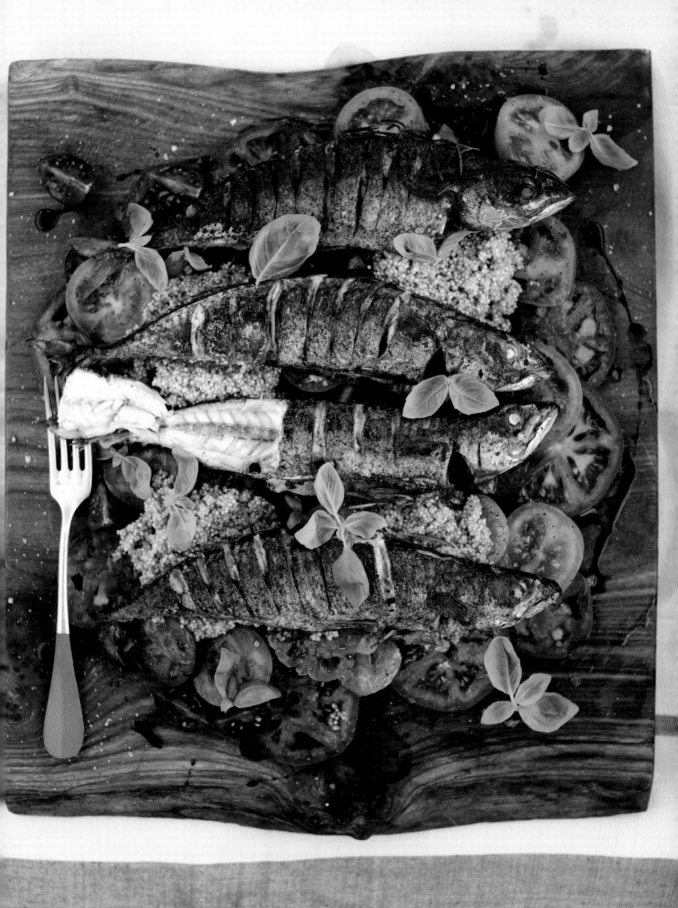

POACHED FISH
CODDLED EGGS & TOMATO LOAF

SERVES 4 | 633 CALORIES

Ingredients out • Kettle boiled • Oven at 200°C/400°F/gas 6
• Food processor (bowl blade) • Large casserole pan, high heat
• Medium pan, medium heat

Eggs
truffle oil
4 large eggs
2 slices of prosciutto
2 tbsp single cream
10g Parmesan cheese

Tomato loaf
1 small seeded loaf (400g)
2 tbsp jarred sun-dried tomatoes
1 clove of garlic
2 tbsp balsamic vinegar
½ a bunch of fresh thyme

Spring greens
4 spring onions
olive oil
1 bunch of asparagus (300g)
1 tsp mint sauce
1 heaped tsp plain flour
300ml semi-skimmed milk
250g frozen petit pois
200g baby spinach

Fish
400g of any undyed smoked white
  fish fillets, scaled and pin-boned
1 lemon

START COOKING

Rub a 16cm baking dish with 1 teaspoon of truffle oil, then crack in the eggs • Tear the prosciutto slices in half and drape over the egg yolks, then drizzle with the cream • Finely grate over the Parmesan, then put in the oven until the eggs are cooked to your liking

Cut deep crisscrosses into the loaf • Throw the sun-dried tomatoes with 1 teaspoon of their oil, the peeled garlic clove and the balsamic into the processor and blitz to a paste • Pick up the paste with the thyme sprigs, then brush, poke and push everything into the cracks in the bread and pop in the oven

Trim and roughly slice the spring onions, then put into the casserole pan with 1 tablespoon of olive oil • Trim the asparagus and add, along with the mint sauce, flour, milk, peas, spinach and a pinch of salt and pepper, then put the lid on and simmer, correcting the seasoning at the end • Pop the fish into the medium pan, cover with boiling water and simmer gently (roughly 6 minutes) • When everything's ready, flake the fish over the veg, then serve with lemon wedges, the coddled eggs and crispy tomato loaf

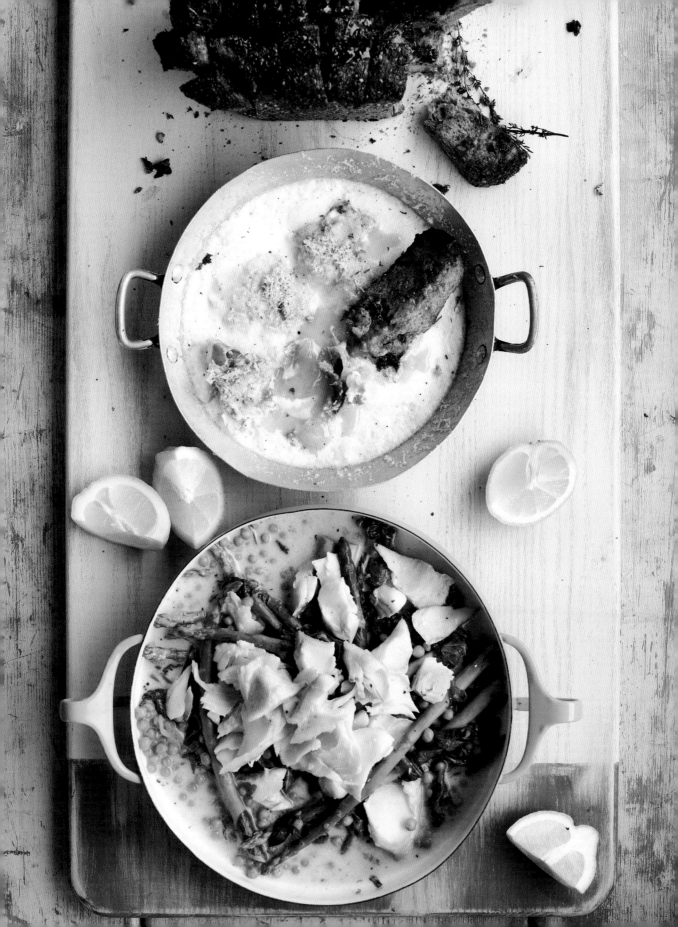

SMOKED SALMON
POTATO & ASPARAGUS SALAD

SERVES 4 | 452 CALORIES

Ingredients out • Kettle boiled • Oven at 160°C/325°F/gas 3
Small lidded pan, high heat • Griddle pan, high heat

Potato & asparagus salad
500g baby new potatoes
4 rashers of smoked pancetta
1 tsp English mustard
1 heaped tsp wholegrain mustard
4 tbsp fat-free natural yoghurt
½ a bunch of fresh dill
white wine vinegar
1 red chicory

Bread
½ a small seeded loaf
unsalted butter

Salmon
240g quality smoked salmon
1 bunch of asparagus (300g)
1 punnet of cress or pea shoots
1 lemon

START COOKING

Halving any larger ones, put the potatoes into the small pan with a pinch of salt, then cover with boiling water and the lid • Pop the bread into the oven • Put the pancetta on the griddle pan, turning when golden, then remove to a board • Lay the smoked salmon over a nice platter in elegant waves, edge to edge

Lay four asparagus spears flat on a board and, holding each one by the stalk end, speed-peel into delicate ribbons (discarding the woody ends), then scatter over the smoked salmon with the snipped cress or pea shoots • Trim the remaining asparagus and throw into the pan with the potatoes, then replace the lid

Put the mustards, yoghurt, chopped dill and a lug of vinegar into a large shallow serving bowl and season to taste • Drain the potatoes and asparagus and toss into the bowl, then finely slice and sprinkle over the chicory and crumble over the crispy pancetta • Serve with bread, a little butter and lemon wedges

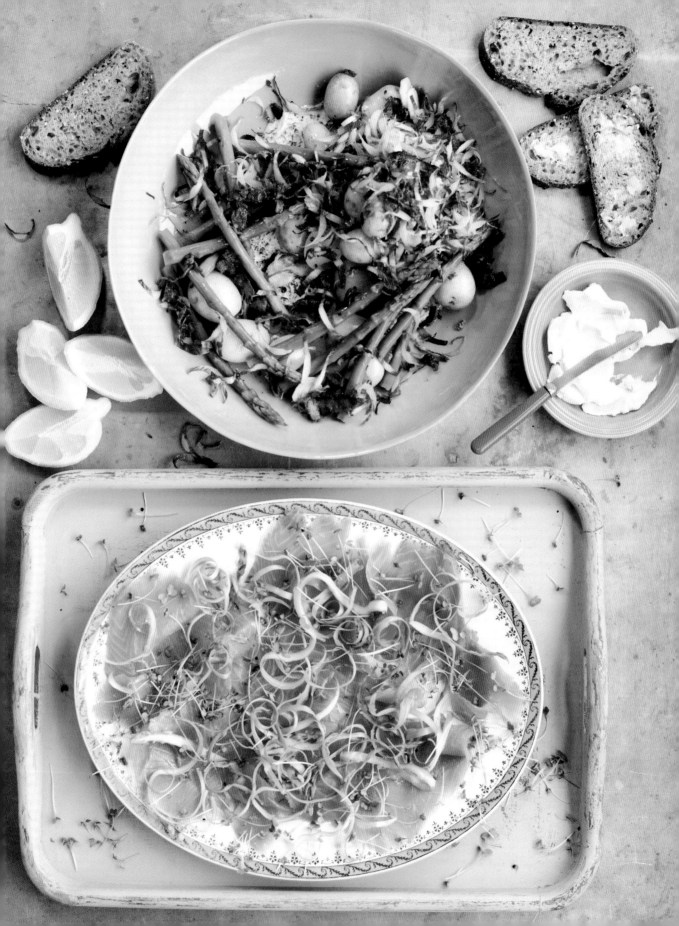

FLASHY FISH STEW
SAFFRON SAUCE & GARLIC BREAD

SERVES 4 | 516 CALORIES

Ingredients out • Kettle boiled • Oven at 220°C/425°F/gas 7
• Food processor (bowl blade) • Large lidded casserole pan, medium heat

Garlic bread
1 ciabatta loaf
3–4 cloves of garlic
a few sprigs of fresh lemon thyme
1 tbsp extra virgin olive oil

Fish stew
1 bulb of fennel
4 anchovy fillets
4 spring onions
½–1 fresh red chilli
olive oil
2 cloves of garlic
125ml white wine
700g passata
1 small bunch of fresh basil
400g mixture of fish fillets,
    scaled and pin-boned. I like
    monkfish, red mullet, John Dory,
    sea bass and whiting
400g mussels and clams, scrubbed
    clean and debearded
4 large raw shell-on king prawns

Sauce
1 clove of garlic
1 pinch of saffron
3 heaped tbsp fat-free natural
    yoghurt
½ a lemon

START COOKING
Cut deep crisscrosses into the ciabatta • Squash the unpeeled garlic through a garlic crusher over the bread, add the thyme sprigs and a pinch of salt and pepper, then drizzle over the extra virgin olive oil • Rub into the cracks of the bread, then put into the oven until golden

Halve the fennel (reserving any leafy tops) and put into the processor with the anchovies, the trimmed spring onions and chilli, then blitz until finely chopped • Put into the casserole pan with 2 tablespoons of olive oil and turn the heat up to high, stirring regularly • Squash in the unpeeled garlic through a garlic crusher, then pour the wine into the pan and let it cook away • Pour in the passata and half a jar of boiling water (350ml), tear in most of the basil leaves and season with salt and pepper

Cut the fish up so you've got four even-sized chunks of each type, then add all the seafood to the pan (throw away any open mussels and clams that don't close when tapped), cover with the lid and boil • Peel the garlic and bash with a pinch of salt and the saffron in a pestle and mortar, then muddle in the yoghurt and a squeeze of lemon juice • When the mussels and clams have opened (throw away any that remain closed), the fish will be cooked through (roughly 4 minutes) • Season to taste, then serve scattered with the remaining basil leaves and fennel tops, the saffron sauce and garlic bread

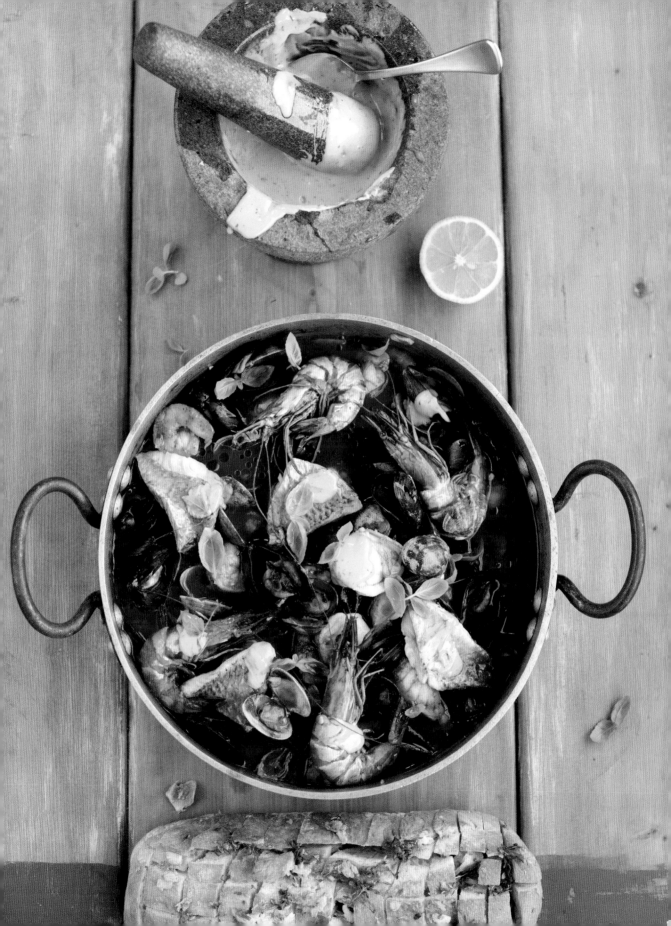

SEARED ASIAN TUNA
COCONUT RICE & JIGGY JIGGY GREENS

Ingredients out • Kettle boiled • Small lidded pan, medium-high heat • Large frying pan, medium-high heat • Food processor (fine slicer)

Rice

1 x 400g tin of light coconut milk
1 coconut milk tin (300g)
    of basmati rice
1 lime

Tuna

1 x 450g piece of yellowfin
    tuna steak
2 green tea bags
1 tbsp sesame seeds
olive oil
1 x 105g packet of pickled ginger
2 spring onions
1 fresh red chilli
1 pink grapefruit
low-salt soy sauce
½ a bunch of fresh coriander

Greens

2 bok choi
1 large bunch of asparagus (300g)
200g tenderstem broccoli
2 tsp sesame oil, plus extra
    to serve
3 cloves of garlic
1 tbsp Teriyaki sauce

START COOKING

Pour the coconut milk, 1 tin's worth of rice and 1 tin of boiling water (use a tea towel) into the small pan • Season with salt and pepper, stir well, cover and cook for roughly 10 minutes, stirring occasionally, then turn the heat off • Halve the tuna lengthways, then empty the contents of the tea bags on to a board with the sesame seeds and a pinch of salt and pepper • Roll and press the tuna in the flavours to coat, then put into the frying pan with 1 tablespoon of olive oil • Sear for about 40 seconds on each side, then remove to a plate, leaving the pan on the heat

Halve the bok choi, then finely slice in the processor with the trimmed asparagus and broccoli • Put the sesame oil into the frying pan and turn the heat up to high • Squash in the unpeeled garlic through a garlic crusher, then tip in the sliced greens • Toss and move around for 2 minutes, then season to taste with Teriyaki sauce and remove from the heat

Pour the pickled ginger and its juices on to a nice serving platter • Finely slice the trimmed spring onions and chilli and sprinkle over the top • Squeeze over the grapefruit juice and season to taste • Slice the tuna 1cm thick and place on the dressing, drizzle with a little soy sauce, then sprinkle with coriander leaves and a few dribbles of sesame oil • Serve with the rice, lime wedges and greens

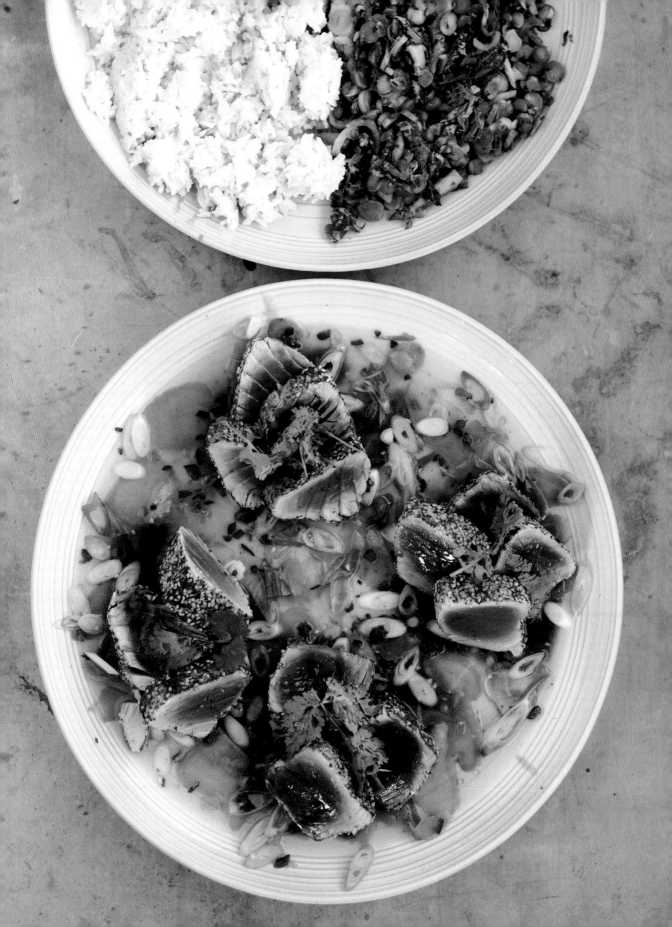

WHITE FISH TAGINE
CARROT, CORIANDER & CLEMENTINE SALAD

Ingredients out • Kettle boiled • High-sided roasting tray, medium heat • Small frying pan, low heat • Food processor (grater)

Couscous
½ a lemon
½ a bunch of fresh mint
1 mug (300g) of couscous

Tagine
olive oil
2 cloves of garlic
1 handful of mixed olives (stone in)
2 tsp harissa
2 anchovy fillets
700g passata
1 small preserved lemon
1 good pinch of saffron
4 x 120g plaice fillets, skin off
  and pin-boned

Salad
2 tbsp sesame seeds
3 medium carrots
3 clementines
1 tbsp extra virgin olive oil
½ a lemon
½ a bunch of fresh coriander

To serve
1 tbsp harissa
4 tbsp fat-free natural yoghurt

START COOKING

Put ½ a lemon, the mint stalks (reserving the top leafy half) and a pinch of salt into a nice serving bowl with 1 mug of couscous and 2 mugs of boiling water, then cover • Drizzle 2 tablespoons of olive oil into the roasting tray and squash in the unpeeled garlic through a garlic crusher • Stir the olives, harissa, anchovies and passata into the tray, and tear in the preserved lemon

Cover the saffron with a splash of boiling water • Season each fish fillet with salt and pepper, roll up and place in the sauce, then sprinkle the fish with the saffron • Scrunch up and wet a sheet of greaseproof paper, tuck it over the fish and leave to simmer fast until cooked through (roughly 8 minutes) • Taste and correct the seasoning • Toast the sesame seeds in the frying pan until golden, then remove

Grate the trimmed carrots in the processor and pile on to a serving plate • Peel the clementines, slice into rounds and place on top, then tear over the mint leaves and drizzle with the extra virgin olive oil and lemon juice • Sprinkle over the toasted sesame seeds, season with salt and pepper and toss together • In a small bowl, marble the harissa through the yoghurt • Fluff up the couscous and serve with the fish tagine and carrot salad, sprinkling everything with coriander leaves

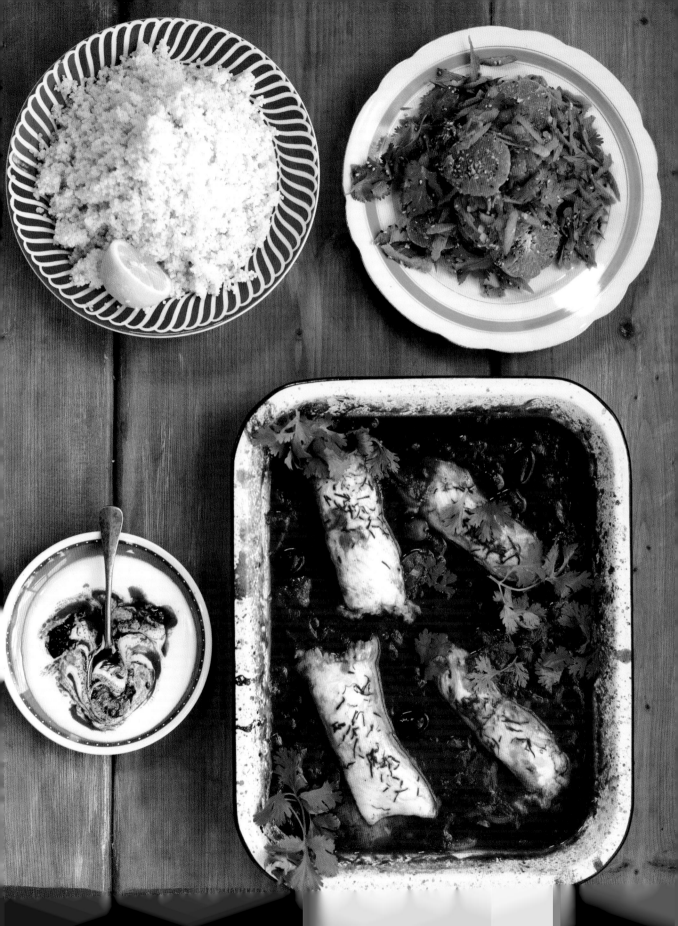

LUCKY SQUID 'N' PRAWNS
SPICY VEGETABLE NOODLE BROTH

SERVES 4 | 446 CALORIES

Broth

2 chicken stock cubes
¼ of a head of cauliflower
1 red pepper
200g sugar snap peas
1 bok choi
4 nests of fine egg noodles
2 limes

Paste

1 thumb-sized piece of ginger
2 cloves of garlic
2 sticks of lemongrass
6 kaffir lime leaves
1 fresh red chilli
1 bunch of fresh coriander
1 tbsp runny honey
1 tbsp fish sauce
1 tbsp low-salt soy sauce,
 plus extra to serve
1 tbsp sesame oil

Seafood

200g squid, gutted and cleaned
200g large raw peeled tiger prawns
140g mixed mushrooms
1 tbsp runny honey

*Ingredients out • Kettle boiled • Medium lidded casserole pan, high heat
• Food processor (bowl blade & thick slicer) • Large griddle pan, high heat*

START COOKING

Pour 1.5 litres of boiling water into the casserole pan and crumble in the stock cubes • Peel the ginger, garlic and the outer leaves of the lemongrass, roughly chop them and put into the processor • Add the lime leaves, chilli, coriander stalks, honey, fish and soy sauces and the sesame oil, then whiz until combined

Put 1 heaped tablespoon of that paste in a bowl, then add the rest to the hot broth • Cut open the squid tubes and using a regular eating knife, lightly score the inside in a 0.5cm crisscross, put into the bowl with the squid legs, prawns and mushrooms, then toss to coat in the paste and put aside • Swap to the thick slicer in the processor and slice the cauliflower, deseeded pepper, sugar snaps and bok choi

Stir the noodles and sliced veg into the broth, put the lid on and bring back to the boil for 2 minutes – don't overcook it • Place the squid and mushrooms on the screaming hot griddle pan, sprinkle over the prawns and cook until lightly charred on both sides, then drizzle with the honey • Season the broth thoughtfully to taste with soy sauce and lime juice, then scatter with the coriander leaves • Slice up the squid and serve

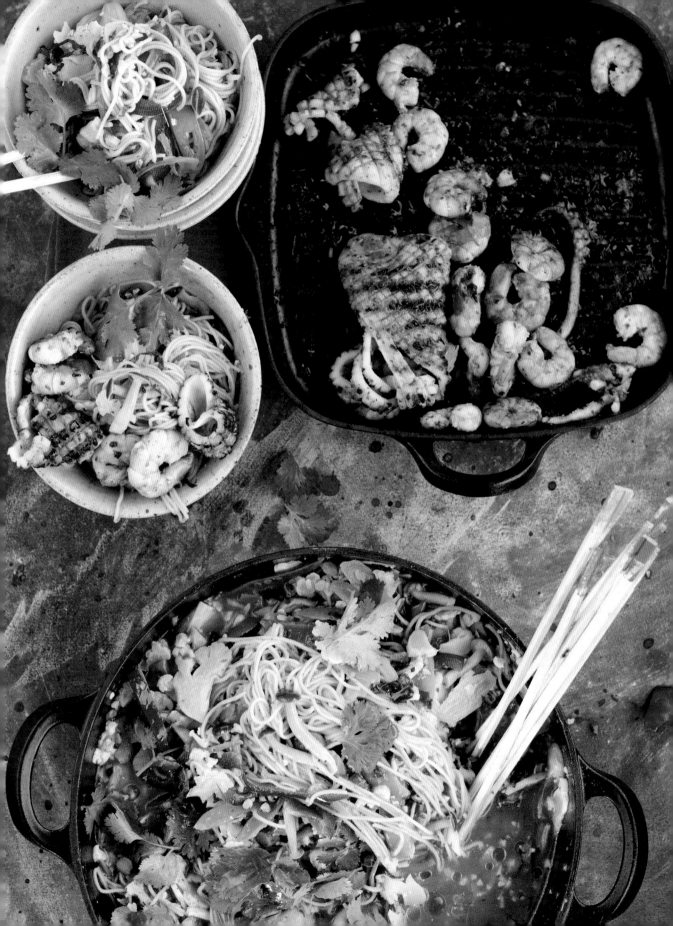

KOH SAMUI SALAD
CHILLI TOFU & THAI NOODLES

Ingredients out • Kettle boiled • Medium frying pan, low heat • Food processor (bowl blade & fine slicer)

Salad

300g medium rice noodles
1 clove of garlic
1 thumb-sized piece of ginger
6 ripe cherry tomatoes
1 fresh red chilli
½ a bunch of fresh basil
1 heaped tsp golden caster sugar
3 tbsp fish sauce
2 tbsp sesame oil
3 limes
1 bunch of radishes
2 carrots
½ a cucumber
1 bulb of fennel
½ a white cabbage
100g cooked peeled prawns

Garnish

100g shelled peanuts
2 tbsp sesame seeds
1 tsp sesame oil
3 dried kaffir lime leaves
1 bunch of fresh mint
350g silken tofu
1 tbsp sweet chilli sauce
1 lime

START COOKING

Put the noodles in a bowl and cover with boiling water, mixing up regularly to separate • In the frying pan, toast the peanuts and sesame seeds with the sesame oil and crumbled lime leaves until golden, tossing often • Put the peeled garlic and ginger, tomatoes, chilli and top leafy half of the basil into the processor with the sugar, fish sauce, sesame oil and juice of 3 limes, then blitz until fine

With the dressing still in the processor, swap to the fine slicer and slice the radishes, trimmed carrots, cucumber, quartered fennel and wedged-up cabbage • Tip it all into a big bowl, scrunch and dress the salad quite roughly with clean hands, then have a taste and tweak the flavours if needed

Drain the noodles, add to the salad bowl with the prawns, and toss together • Rip off the top leafy half of the mint, roughly chop it and scatter over the top • Cut the tofu into 2cm chunks and pile in the middle of the salad drizzled with chilli sauce • Scatter over the toasted nuts and serve with lime wedges

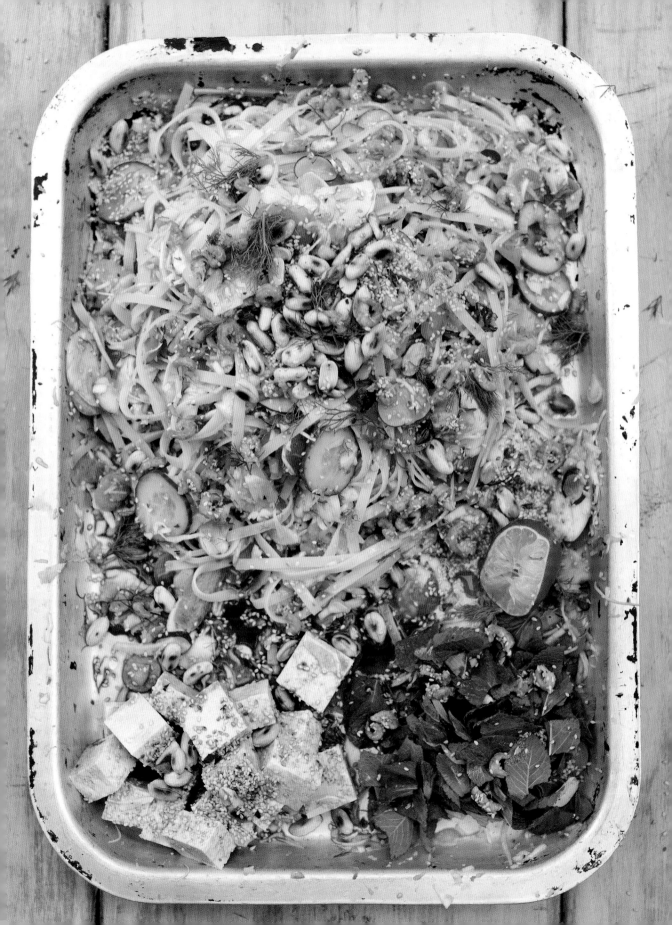

BUTTERFLIED SARDINES TUSCAN BREAD SALAD

SERVES 4 | 399 CALORIES

Ingredients out • Oven grill on high • Food processor (bowl blade) • Griddle pan, high heat

Sardines

1 pinch of saffron
4 spring onions
½ a fresh red chilli
½ a bunch of fresh flat-leaf parsley
½ tsp fennel seeds
2 lemons
olive oil
8 fresh sardines, scaled
    and butterflied
4 rashers of smoked pancetta

Salad

½ a ciabatta loaf
1 clove of garlic
4 anchovy fillets
extra virgin olive oil
3 tbsp balsamic vinegar
800g ripe mixed-colour tomatoes
½ a bunch of spring onions
½ a bunch of fresh basil
1 tbsp capers
200g jarred roasted red peppers
30g feta cheese

START COOKING

Put the saffron, trimmed spring onions, chilli, parsley, fennel seeds, juice of 1 lemon, 1 tablespoon of olive oil, and a pinch of salt and pepper into the processor, then pulse to a coarse paste • Rub the paste over a baking tray just big enough to lay out the sardines flat on top, skin side up • Lay the pancetta in waves between the fish, then grill until golden and crispy (roughly 8 minutes)

Cut four 2cm-thick slices of ciabatta and place on the griddle pan until toasted on both sides • Peel the garlic and put into the processor with the anchovies, 1 tablespoon of extra virgin olive oil, the balsamic and half the tomatoes, trimmed spring onions and basil • Whiz to a smooth dressing and season nicely to taste, then tip into a large serving bowl

Add the capers to the bowl, then randomly cut up and add the peppers • Tear the ciabatta into thumb-sized pieces, add to the bowl and toss together • Halve or quarter the remaining tomatoes, trim and finely slice the remaining spring onions and add, then pick over the rest of the basil leaves • Crumble over the feta, and drizzle with 1 teaspoon of extra virgin olive oil to finish • Serve with the sardines and lemon wedges

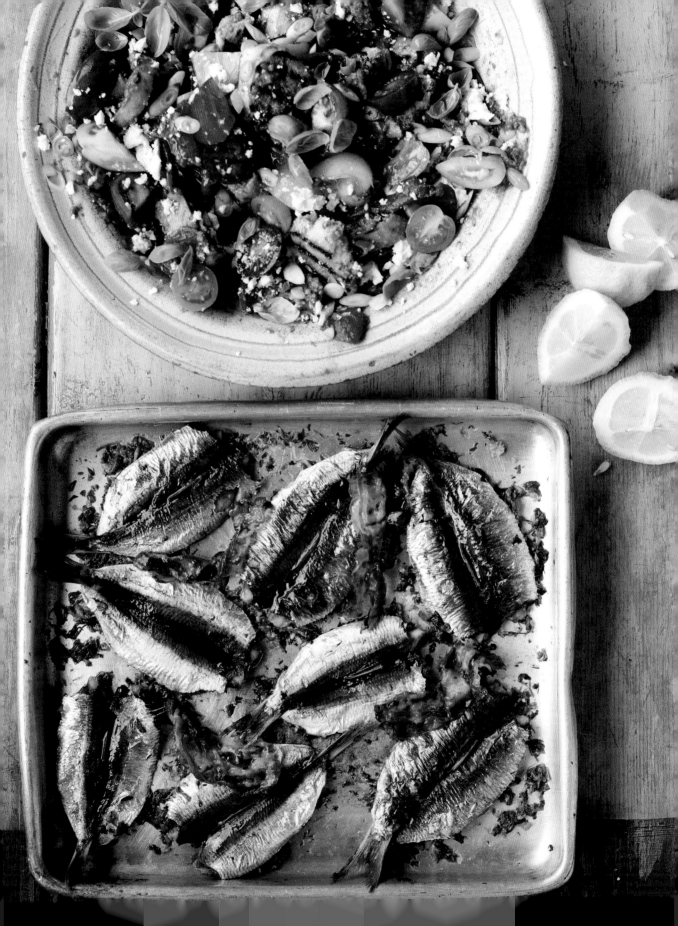

CHORIZO & SQUID
GREEK-STYLE COUSCOUS SALAD

SERVES 4 | 634 CALORIES

Ingredients out • Kettle boiled • Food processor (bowl blade)
• Large frying pan, high heat

Couscous
4 spring onions
100g baby spinach
1 bunch of fresh mint
1 mug (300g) of couscous
1 lemon

Chorizo & squid
400g baby squid, gutted
  and cleaned
80g cured chorizo sausage
olive oil
2 mixed-colour peppers
1 tbsp runny honey
sherry vinegar
2 cloves of garlic
8–10 black olives (stone in)

Garnishes
50g feta cheese
1 heaped tsp harissa
4 tbsp fat-free natural yoghurt

START COOKING

Blitz the trimmed spring onions in the processor with the spinach, most of the top leafy half of the mint and a pinch of salt and pepper until fine • Remove the blade, stir in 1 mug of couscous and 2 mugs of boiling water, put the lid on and leave to sit in the processor • Cut open the squid tubes and, using a regular eating knife, lightly score the inside in 0.5cm crisscrosses, then slice with a sharp knife about 1cm thick, and roughly slice the legs

Slice the chorizo and put it into the pan with 2 tablespoons of oil • Deseed, slice and add the peppers, then about 4 minutes later stir in all the squid, the honey and a splash of vinegar • Squash over the unpeeled garlic through a garlic crusher, destone and add the olives and stir for a few more minutes

Fluff up the couscous and mix with the juice of ½ a lemon, then tip on to a big board or platter • Spoon the squid, peppers and chorizo over the couscous • Crumble the feta over the top and pick over the remaining mint leaves • In a small bowl, ripple the harissa through the yoghurt and serve everything together, with lemon wedges on the side

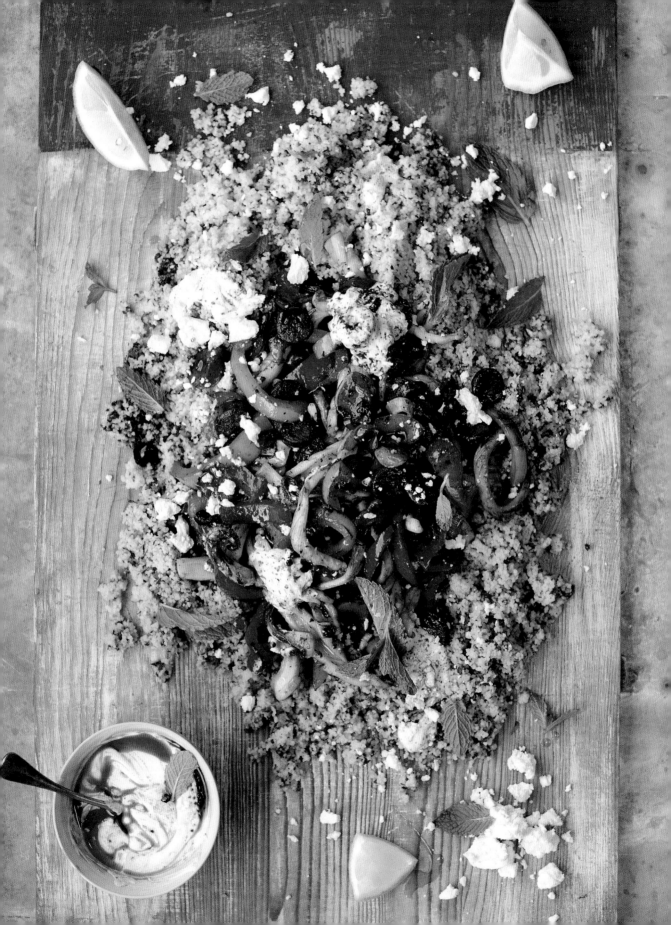

BAKED WHOLE TROUT
JERSEY ROYALS, PEAS & MUSTARD SAUCE

SERVES 4 | 504 CALORIES

Ingredients out • Kettle boiled • Oven at full whack (240°C/475°F/gas 9) • Food processor (thick slicer) • Lidded casserole pan, high heat

Trout

4 x 250g trout, scaled and gutted
olive oil
1 lemon
1 bunch of fresh thyme
40g flaked almonds
4 rashers of smoked pancetta

Veg

600g new potatoes
2 chicken stock cubes
2 little gem lettuces
1 bunch of fresh mint
300g frozen peas
200g frozen broad beans

Sauce

2 tsp jarred grated horseradish
1 tsp English mustard
½ a lemon
4 tbsp fat-free natural yoghurt

START COOKING

On a baking tray, season the trout with salt, pepper and 1 tablespoon of oil • Cut the lemon into quarters, add to the tray and cook on the top shelf of the oven • Slice the new potatoes in the processor and put into the casserole pan with 1 litre of boiling water • Crumble in the stock cubes, cover with the lid and boil

In a bowl, mix the horseradish, mustard, juice from ½ a lemon and a small pinch of salt together, then ripple it through the yoghurt • Slice up the gem lettuces and finely chop the top leafy half of the mint

Toss the thyme sprigs in 1 teaspoon of oil, then scatter over the trout with the flaked almonds • Lay a piece of pancetta over each fish and put back into the oven for a few minutes, until golden and crispy • Stir the lettuce, mint leaves, peas and broad beans into the potato pan • Season to taste, cook for a couple of minutes, then serve with the crispy trout and mustard sauce

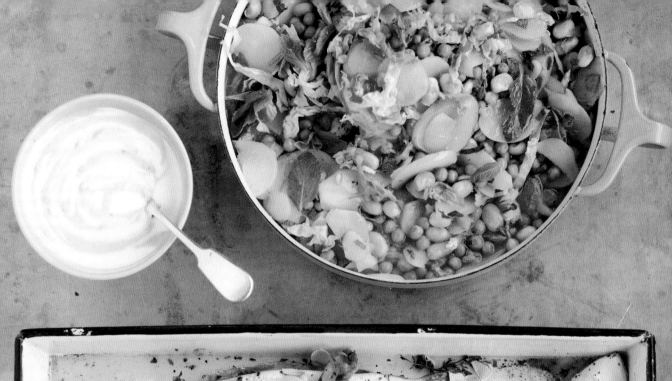
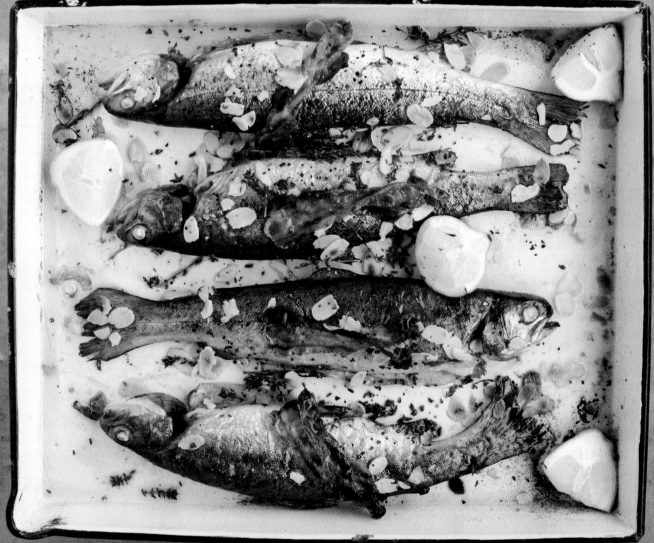

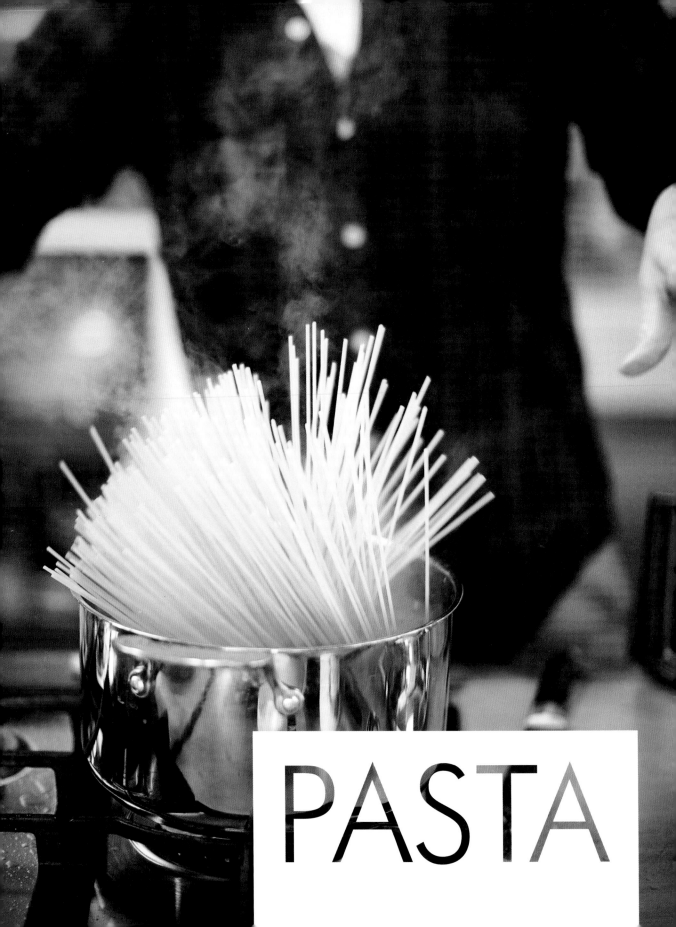

PASTA

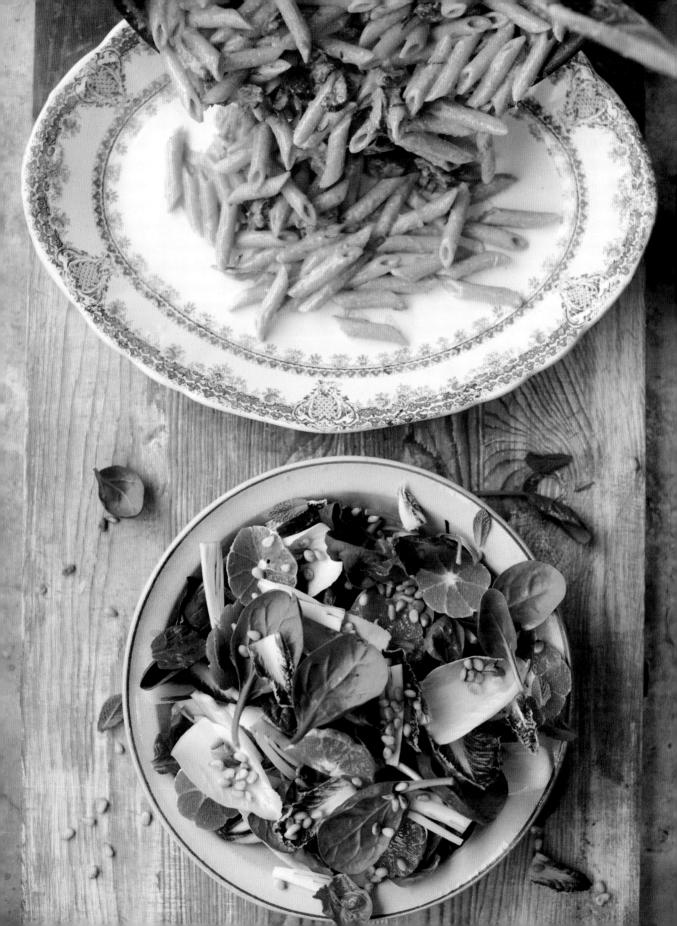

PASTA PESTO
GARLIC & ROSEMARY CHICKEN

SERVES 4 | 581 CALORIES

Ingredients out • Kettle boiled • Large frying pan, high heat
• Large lidded casserole pan, high heat • Food processor (bowl blade)

Chicken

2 x 200g skinless chicken breasts
1 tsp fennel seeds
2 sprigs of fresh rosemary
2 tbsp rapeseed oil
4–5 cloves of garlic
1–2 fresh red chillies
8 ripe cherry tomatoes

Pasta & pesto

250g green beans
1 big bunch of fresh basil
50g blanched almonds
50g Parmesan cheese,
   plus extra to serve
2 tbsp extra virgin olive oil
1 lemon
1 clove of garlic
300g fresh lasagne sheets
200g baby spinach

START COOKING

On a large sheet of greaseproof paper, toss the chicken with salt, pepper, fennel seeds and the rosemary leaves • Fold over the paper, then bash and flatten the chicken to 1.5cm thick with a rolling pin • Put into the frying pan with the rapeseed oil, the bashed unpeeled garlic cloves and halved chillies, turning after about 3 or 4 minutes, until golden and cooked through • Line the beans up and cut off the stalks, put into the casserole pan, cover with boiling salted water and cook for 6 minutes with the lid on

Pick a few basil leaves for garnish, then rip off the stalks and put the rest of the bunch into the processor with the almonds, Parmesan, extra virgin olive oil and lemon juice • Squash in the unpeeled garlic through a garlic crusher • Blitz until smooth, adding a ladle or two of cooking water from the beans to loosen, then season to taste • Slice the lasagne sheets up into random handkerchief shapes and add to the beans to cook for a couple of minutes • Halve or quarter the tomatoes, add to the chicken and give the pan a shake

Stir the spinach into the pasta pan, then drain, reserving a cupful of the starchy cooking water • Return the pasta, beans and spinach to the pan, pour in the pesto from the processor and stir together, loosening with splashes of cooking water until silky • Slice the chicken breasts in half and serve with the tomatoes and chilli spooned over the top • Finely grate a little extra Parmesan over the pasta, then sprinkle everything with basil leaves

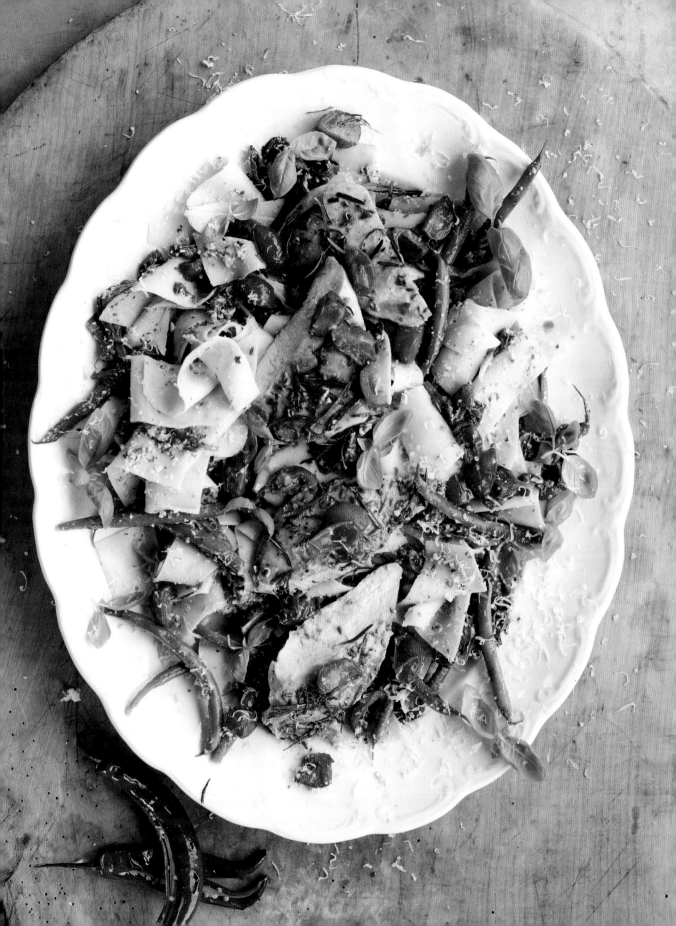

CRAB BOLOGNESE
CRUNCHY FENNEL SALAD

SERVES 4 | 673 CALORIES

Ingredients out • Kettle boiled • Food processor (bowl blade & fine slicer)
• Lidded casserole pan, medium heat • Large lidded pan, high heat

Pasta & sauce
½–1 fresh red chilli
1 carrot
2 spring onions
2 cloves of garlic
1 heaped tsp fennel seeds
2 anchovy fillets
½ a bunch of fresh basil
2 bulbs of fennel
olive oil
320g dried spaghetti
1 lemon
300g crabmeat
   (brown and white meat)
white wine
700g passata

Salad
2 little gem lettuces
½ a bunch of fresh mint
1 lemon
Parmesan cheese
1 tbsp extra virgin olive oil

START COOKING

Halve the chilli, carrot and trimmed spring onions and put them in the processor with the peeled garlic, fennel seeds, anchovies and basil stalks • Chop off and add the top stalky part of the fennel, reserving the bulbs (and any leafy tops), then blitz everything until finely chopped • Tip into the casserole pan with 1 tablespoon of olive oil, stirring often • Put the spaghetti into the large pan, cover with boiling salted water and cook according to packet instructions

Finely grate the lemon zest over the veg • Add the brown crabmeat, a splash of white wine and the passata, then stir, cover and leave to simmer • Swap to the fine slicer in the processor • Halve the fennel bulbs and trim the lettuces, then slice them in the processor and tip into a salad bowl • Rip off and slice the top leafy half of the mint, and add to the bowl with a pinch of salt and pepper, the juice of 1 lemon and a few shavings of Parmesan

Roughly chop the top leafy half of the basil and sprinkle most of it into the sauce with the white crabmeat, then squeeze in the juice of the zested lemon • Loosen the sauce with a little starchy cooking water from the spaghetti, then drain the spaghetti and tip into a large bowl • Spoon the sauce on top and serve right away, scattered with the reserved basil leaves, mixing at the table, with the crunchy fennel salad on the other side, finishing both with a drizzle of extra virgin olive oil

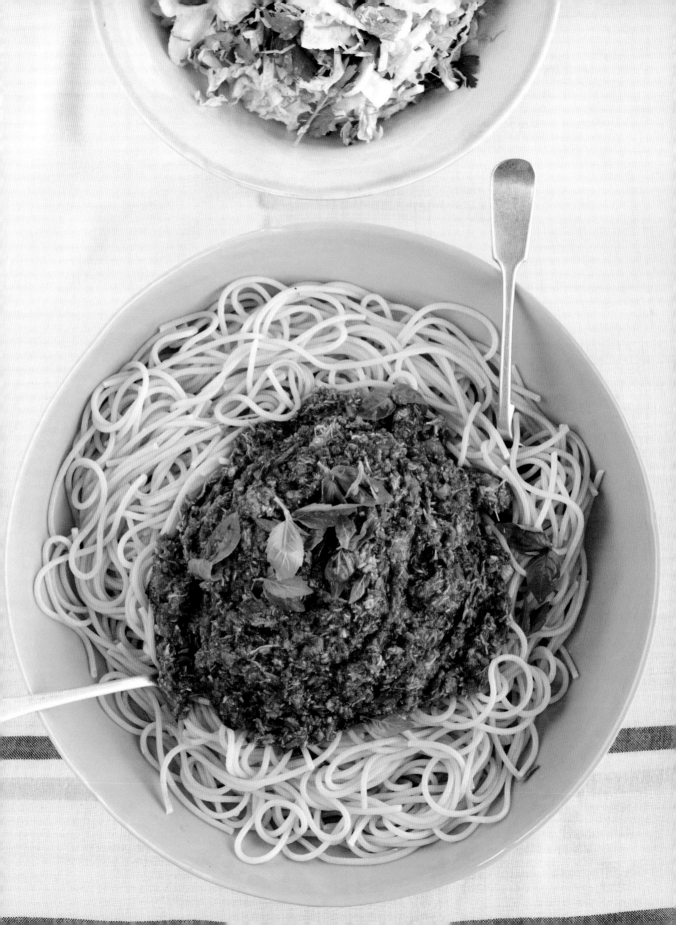

SAUSAGE FUSILLI
CREAMY GARDEN SALAD

Ingredients out • *Kettle boiled* • *Griddle pan, high heat* • *Food processor (bowl blade)* • *Large frying pan, high heat* • *Large lidded pan, high heat*

Pasta

4 sausages (at least 80% meat)
olive oil
1 large red onion
1 heaped tsp fennel seeds
4 jarred red peppers
4 sprigs of fresh rosemary
4 cloves of garlic
320g dried fusilli
3 tbsp thick balsamic vinegar,
   plus extra to serve
350g passata

Salad

1 soft round lettuce
100g baby spinach or rocket
1 punnet of cress
2 tsp English mustard
3 tbsp fat-free natural yoghurt
1 lemon
1 bunch of fresh chives

START COOKING

Score the sausages lengthways about three-quarters of the way through, open them out like a book, then rub with 1 teaspoon of oil and place on the griddle pan, cut side down, turning regularly, until crispy and cooked through • Peel and halve the red onion, then pulse in the processor with the fennel seeds, peppers, half of the rosemary leaves and a pinch of salt and pepper • Put into the large frying pan with 1 tablespoon of oil, squash in the unpeeled garlic through a garlic crusher and stir frequently

Put the pasta into the lidded pan, cover with boiling salted water and cook according to packet instructions • Add the balsamic and passata to the veg pan • Trim the lettuce and cut into wedges, then arrange with the spinach or rocket around a nice board or platter and snip over the cress • Toss the remaining rosemary leaves with the sausages until crispy, then remove from the heat

Make a dressing by mixing the mustard, yoghurt and lemon juice with a pinch of salt and pepper • Finely chop the chives, stir half through the dressing, then drizzle over the salad • Drain the pasta, reserving a cupful of the starchy cooking water, then toss well with the sauce, loosening with a splash of cooking water, if needed • Season to taste and tip on to a platter, scatter over the remaining chives, chop and scatter over the sausages and finish with a drizzle of balsamic from a height

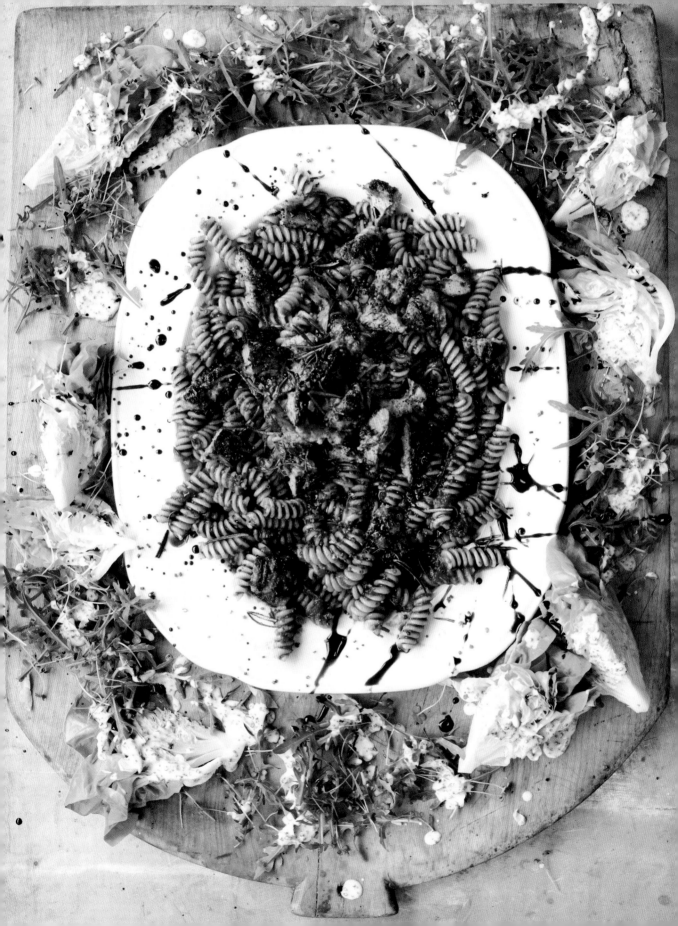

CHORIZO CARBONARA
CATALAN MARKET SALAD

SERVES 4 | 603 CALORIES

Ingredients out • Kettle boiled • Large frying pan, medium heat
• Large lidded pan, high heat

Salad

25g pine nuts
1 red chicory
1 green chicory
2 clementines
100g baby spinach
4 sprigs of fresh mint
45g Manchego cheese
2 tbsp sherry vinegar
2 tbsp extra virgin olive oil
1 tsp runny honey

Pasta

320g dried penne
70g chorizo
½–1 fresh red chilli
2 sprigs of fresh rosemary
olive oil
4 cloves of garlic
1 large egg
½ a lemon
2 heaped tbsp fat-free
    natural yoghurt

START COOKING

Toast the pine nuts in the frying pan for a few minutes, tossing often • Put the pasta into the lidded pan, cover with boiling salted water and cook according to packet instructions • Finely slice the stalk ends of the chicory and click apart the upper leaves into a serving bowl • Peel and finely slice the clementines, add to the bowl with the baby spinach, then pick over the mint leaves • Shave over a tiny bit of Manchego and scatter with the hot nuts, returning the frying pan to a medium heat

In a cup, make your dressing with the vinegar, extra virgin olive oil and honey, then season to taste and put aside • Finely slice the chorizo, chilli and rosemary leaves and put into the frying pan with 1 teaspoon of olive oil and a pinch of pepper, then squash in the unpeeled garlic through a garlic crusher and move everything around until lightly golden

Beat the egg, lemon juice, yoghurt and remaining finely grated Manchego together in a bowl • Drain the pasta, reserving a cupful of the starchy cooking water • Toss the pasta into the chorizo pan, remove from the heat and mix well with the creamy sauce, loosening with a splash of cooking water, if needed, then season to taste • Dress and toss the salad, then serve with the pasta

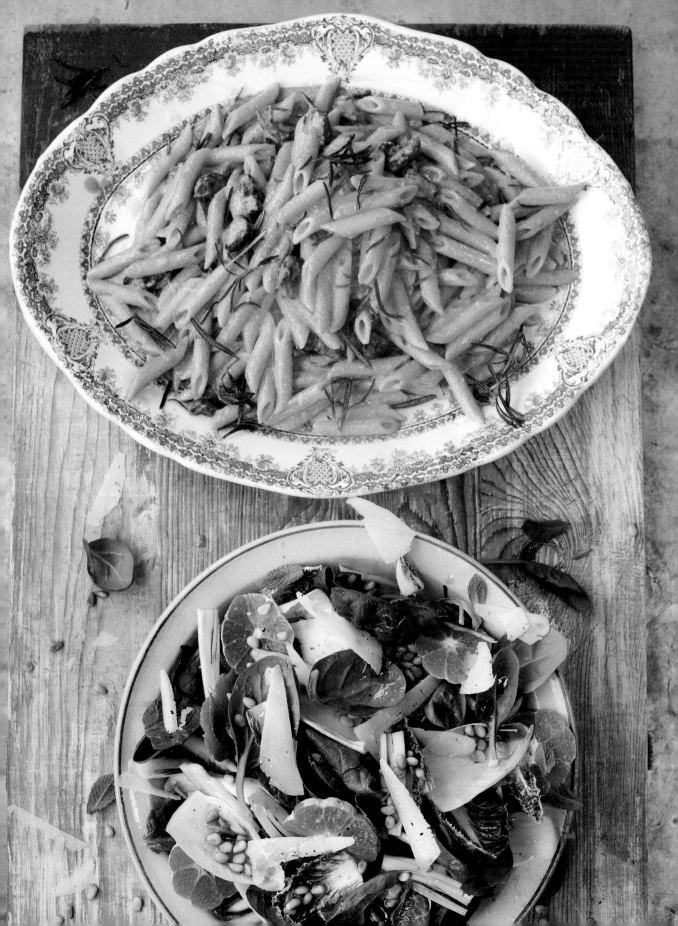

WINTER SQUASH PENNE
MINT & AVOCADO CHOPPED SALAD

SERVES 4 | 635 CALORIES

Ingredients out • Kettle boiled • Food processor (bowl blade) • Lidded casserole pan, medium heat • Large lidded pan, high heat • Stick blender

Pasta

1 vegetable stock cube
1 butternut squash (neck end only)
1 onion
1 tsp fennel seeds
1 small dried red chilli
½ a bunch of fresh sage
1 x 400g tin of chickpeas
320g dried penne
20g Parmesan cheese,
    plus extra to serve
½ a bunch of fresh flat-leaf parsley

Salad

3 ripe tomatoes
½ a cucumber
4 spring onions
2 little gem lettuces
½ a bunch of fresh mint
1 ripe avocado
2 tbsp extra virgin olive oil
2 tbsp balsamic vinegar
20g feta cheese

START COOKING

Make 500ml of hot stock with the cube, then refill and boil the kettle • Trim the stalk off the squash, roughly chop the neck end (don't peel, and keep the seed end for another day), then blitz in the processor with the peeled onion, fennel seeds, dried chilli and sage leaves until combined • Put into the casserole pan, add the stock, chickpeas and their juice, then put the lid on and stir regularly

Put the pasta into the large pan, cover with boiling salted water and cook according to packet instructions • On a large board, chop and mix up the tomatoes, cucumber, trimmed spring onions, lettuce and the top leafy half of the mint • Squeeze and squidge over the avocado, discarding the skin and stone • Dress and toss with the extra virgin olive oil and balsamic, then season to taste and crumble over the feta

Using a stick blender, blitz the sauce to your liking, season well to taste and finely grate in the Parmesan • Drain the pasta, toss with the sauce and season to taste • Serve scattered with chopped parsley leaves and an extra grating of Parmesan

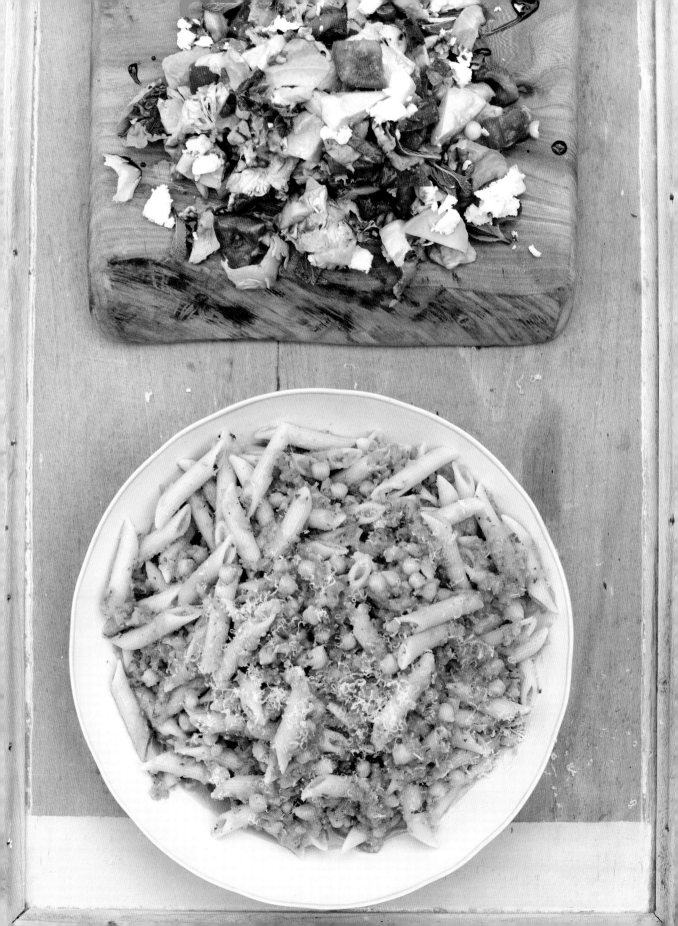

SIMPLE SPAGHETTI
TOMATO, BASIL & CREAMY CURD SALAD

SERVES 4 | 553 CALORIES

Ingredients out • Kettle boiled • Large lidded pan, high heat • Large roasting tray, low heat

Pasta

320g dried spaghetti
300g tenderstem broccoli
½–1 fresh red chilli
8 anchovy fillets
4 cloves of garlic
2 sprigs of fresh rosemary
1 lemon
optional: Parmesan cheese

Salad

500g ripe mixed-colour tomatoes
a few sprigs of fresh basil
extra virgin olive oil
1 tbsp balsamic vinegar
1 lemon
125g low-fat cottage cheese

START COOKING

Put the pasta into the large pan, cover with boiling salted water and cook according to packet instructions • Roughly chop the tomatoes and put them into a bowl • Tear in most of the basil leaves, add 1 tablespoon of oil and the balsamic, then toss and season to taste • Grate the zest of 1 lemon into a nice smallish serving bowl, then squeeze in half the juice • Stir in the cottage cheese, then top with your dressed tomatoes and a few small basil leaves

Trim the broccoli and halve the stalks lengthways, then finely slice the chilli • Turn the heat under the tray up to medium-high and add 4 tablespoons of oil, the chilli and anchovies • Squash in the unpeeled garlic through a garlic crusher, strip in the rosemary leaves and add the broccoli, then add a splash of pasta water • Use tongs to shake and move everything around

Drain the pasta, reserving a cupful of the starchy cooking water, then toss the pasta with the broccoli, the juice of a lemon and enough cooking water to make it shiny • Season to taste, and serve with a grating of Parmesan, if you like, and the tomato, basil and creamy curd salad on the side

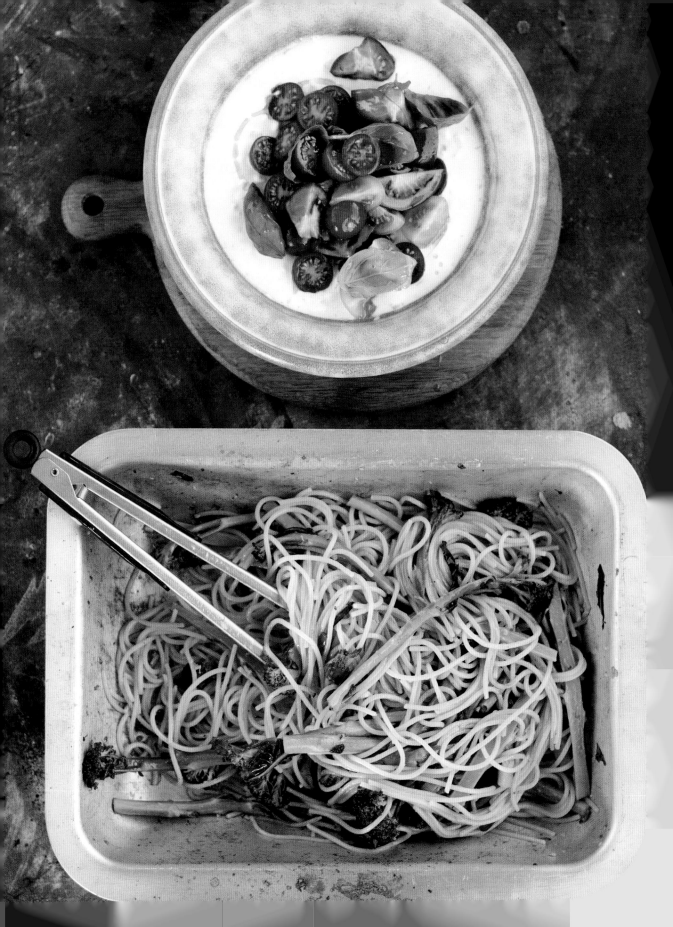

SAUSAGE GNOCCHI
WARM KALE & BEAN SALAD

SERVES 4 | 526 CALORIES

Ingredients out • Kettle boiled • Large casserole pan, high heat • Small frying pan, high heat • Large lidded pan, high heat • Food processor (thick slicer)

Gnocchi

4 spicy sausages
  (at least 80% meat)
2 tsp fennel seeds
2 sprigs of fresh rosemary
125ml Chianti
200g tenderstem broccoli
700g passata
400g gnocchi
2 tbsp fat-free natural yoghurt

Greens

2 rashers of smoked streaky bacon
olive oil
40g blanched hazelnuts
1 tsp maple syrup or runny honey
200g fine green beans
300g mixed greens, such as curly
  kale, Swiss chard, cavolo nero,
  spring greens and Brussels tops
1½ tbsp extra virgin olive oil
1½ tbsp sherry vinegar

START COOKING

Squeeze the sausage meat out of the skins into the casserole pan with the fennel seeds and rosemary leaves (discard the sausage skins) • Break the meat apart, stirring regularly • Finely slice the bacon, put into the small frying pan with 1 teaspoon of olive oil and the hazelnuts and cook until golden, then add the maple syrup or honey and remove from the heat

Line the beans up and cut off the stalks, then put them into the large pan, cover with boiling salted water and the lid • Cook for 4 minutes, then add the greens, tearing up any larger leaves • Pour the wine into the sausage pan and let it bubble away while you check on the beans and greens • If done, use a slotted spoon to transfer them to a colander to drain, leaving the pan of water on the heat • Tear the broccoli tips into the sausage pan, then slice and add the stalks, along with the passata

Add the gnocchi to the pan of water the greens were cooked in and pop the lid on • Mix the extra virgin olive oil, vinegar and a pinch of salt and pepper in a serving bowl, tip in the drained greens and toss to coat, then scatter over the crispy nuts and bacon • When the gnocchi have been floating for a couple of minutes, drain them and toss with the sauce • Season to taste and serve in the pan, or on a nice platter, drizzled with yoghurt

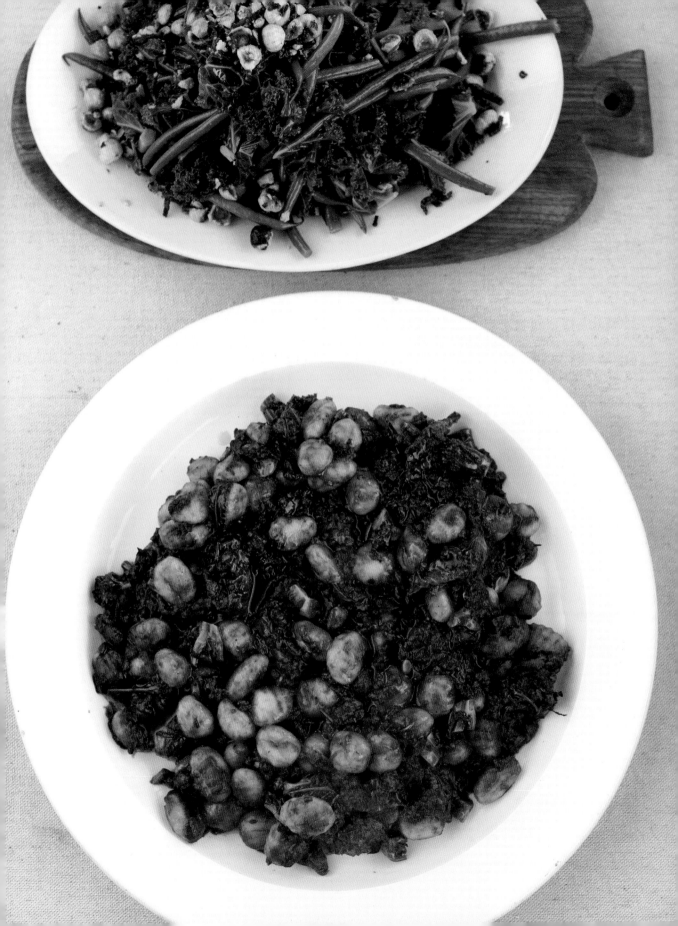

CHICKEN CACCIATORE
SPAGHETTI & SMOKY TOMATO SAUCE

Ingredients out • Kettle boiled • Large frying pan, medium heat • Large lidded pan, medium heat

Chicken & sauce

4 skinless, boneless chicken thighs
olive oil
125g oyster mushrooms
125g chestnut mushrooms
4 rashers of smoked pancetta
2–3 sprigs of fresh rosemary
2 anchovy fillets
2 jarred red peppers
1 small handful of black olives
   (stone in)
2 cloves of garlic
1 fresh red chilli
60ml Chianti
700g passata
1 bunch of fresh basil

Pasta

320g dried wholewheat spaghetti
30g Parmesan cheese

START COOKING

Cut the chicken into 1cm chunks, then put into the large frying pan with 2 tablespoons of oil and a pinch of salt and pepper • Roughly chop the mushrooms, finely slice the pancetta, then add both to the pan with the rosemary leaves, anchovies and torn-up peppers • Squash and add the olives (discarding the stones), then turn the heat up to medium-high, tossing regularly until golden

Put the pasta into the large pan, cover with boiling salted water and cook according to packet instructions • Squash the unpeeled garlic through a garlic crusher into the chicken pan • Finely slice and add the chilli, pour in the wine and passata, then season to taste • Tear in and stir through most of the top leafy half of the basil

Finely grate the Parmesan • Drain the pasta, reserving a cupful of the starchy cooking water, then tip on to a platter and spoon over the sauce • Scatter with the remaining basil leaves and the grated Parmesan • Toss together, loosening with a splash of cooking water, if needed

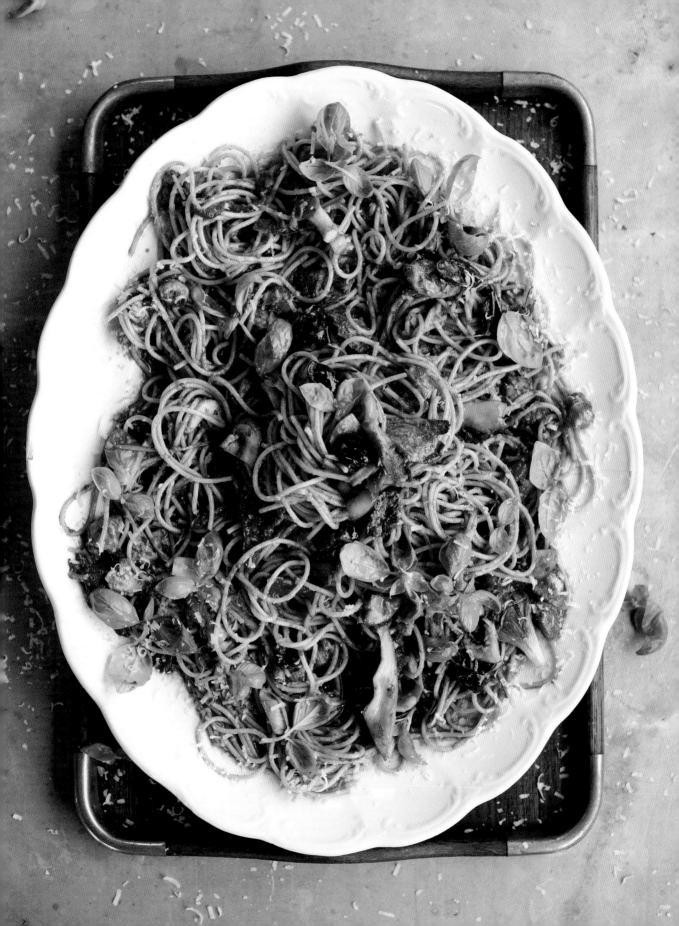

FETTUCCINE
SMOKED TROUT, ASPARAGUS & PEAS

Ingredients out • Kettle boiled • Medium pan, high heat
• Large lidded pan, high heat • Stick blender

Pasta
1 small bunch of spring onions
1 bunch of asparagus (300g)
olive oil
300g frozen peas
1 big bunch of fresh mint
1 tbsp plain flour
500ml semi-skimmed milk
320g dried fettuccine
250g hot-smoked trout
Parmesan cheese, to serve

Salad & dressing
1 red chicory
1 green chicory
1 little gem lettuce
a few sprigs of fresh tarragon
2 heaped tsp Dijon mustard
1 heaped tsp runny honey
1 tbsp extra virgin olive oil
1 lemon
1 heaped tbsp fat-free
   natural yoghurt

START COOKING

Roughly slice the trimmed spring onions and asparagus stalks, leaving the tips whole, and put into the medium pan with 2 tablespoons of olive oil and the peas • Roughly chop most of the top leafy half of the mint, and add it to the pan • Stir in the flour, pour in the milk and bring to the boil, then simmer • Put the pasta into the large pan, cover with boiling salted water and cook according to packet instructions

Cut the chicory and lettuce into long thin wedges and put these into a salad bowl • Pick over the tarragon and the remaining mint leaves • Spoon the mustard and honey into a small bowl, add the extra virgin olive oil, the juice of ½ a lemon and the yoghurt, mix together and season to taste

Using the stick blender, purée the asparagus sauce until fairly smooth • Turn the heat down to low, flake in the trout, add the asparagus tips and simmer for a few more minutes, then squeeze in the rest of the lemon juice and season to taste • Drain the pasta, reserving a cupful of starchy cooking water, then toss the pasta with the sauce, loosening with a splash of cooking water, if needed • Serve straight away, with a grating of Parmesan and the salad, dressing it at the table

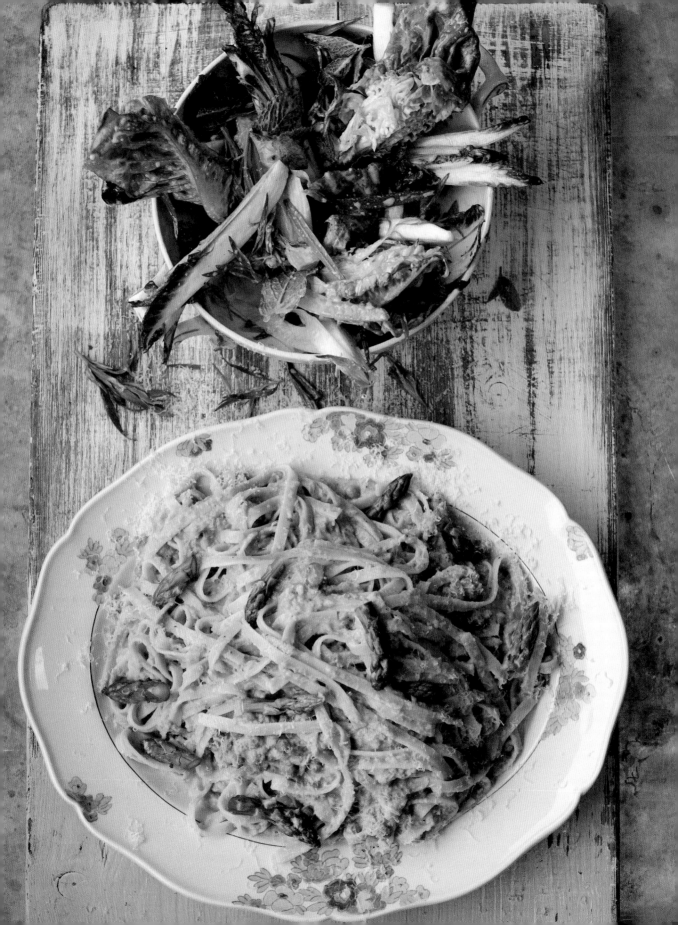

CHICKEN PASTA
HERBY 6-VEG RAGÙ

SERVES 4 | 620 CALORIES

Ingredients out • Kettle boiled • Food processor (bowl blade) • Large casserole pan, high heat • Large lidded pan, medium heat • Medium frying pan, high heat

Ragù

1 large leek
1 stick of celery
1 carrot
1 courgette
3 jarred red peppers
olive oil
8 sprigs of fresh thyme
700g passata

Pasta

320g dried wholewheat fusilli
2 x 150g skinless chicken breasts
3 rashers of smoked streaky bacon
½ a fresh red chilli
4 cloves of garlic
2 sprigs of fresh rosemary
2 fresh bay leaves
1 tbsp pine nuts
balsamic vinegar
Parmesan cheese, to serve

START COOKING

Split the leek lengthways, rinse under the cold tap, then finely chop in the processor with the trimmed celery and carrot, the courgette and peppers • Put into the casserole pan with 1 tablespoon of oil, the thyme leaves and a pinch of salt and pepper and stir regularly • Put the pasta into the large pan, cover with boiling salted water and cook according to packet instructions

Dice the chicken into 2cm chunks and put into the frying pan with 1 tablespoon of oil and a pinch of salt and pepper, tossing regularly until golden and cooked through • Stir the passata into the vegetables and simmer • Finely slice the bacon and chilli and add to the golden chicken, then squash in the unpeeled garlic through a garlic crusher • Strip in the rosemary leaves, add the bay leaves and pine nuts, and fry for a minute or two, until the bacon is golden, then drizzle with balsamic

Season the sauce, drain the pasta, reserving a cupful of starchy cooking water, then toss the pasta with the sauce, loosening with the cooking water, if needed, and pour on to a platter • Scatter the chicken and bacon on top of the pasta and serve with a grating of Parmesan

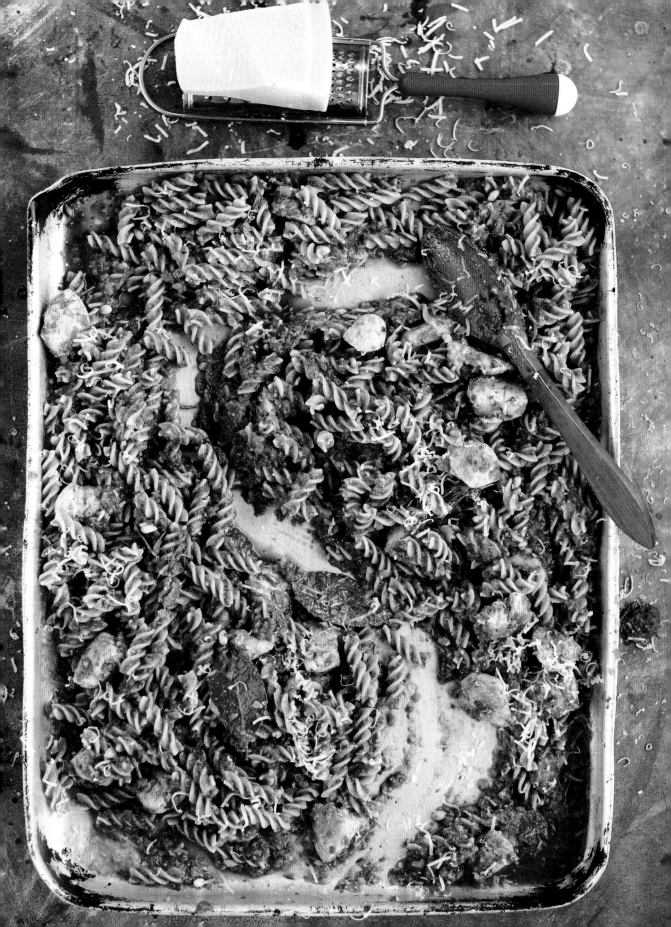

BROCCOLI PASTA
CHOPPED GARDEN SALAD

Ingredients out • *Kettle boiled* • *Large lidded casserole pan, high heat*
• *Liquidizer* • *Small frying pan, low heat*

Pasta

320g dried orecchiette
1 bunch of fresh basil
1 x 50g tin of anchovy
   fillets in oil
1 lemon
2 cloves of garlic
1 dried red chilli
30g Parmesan cheese,
   plus extra to serve
1 large head of broccoli
50g pine nuts

Salad

2 carrots
1 ripe avocado
3 ripe mixed-colour tomatoes
2 tbsp extra virgin olive oil
2 tbsp balsamic vinegar
70g rocket

START COOKING

Put the pasta into the casserole pan, cover with boiling salted water and cook according to packet instructions • Put the basil, anchovies and 1 tablespoon of their oil, the zest and juice of 1 lemon and a splash of boiling water into the liquidizer • Squash in the unpeeled garlic through a garlic crusher, crumble in the dried chilli, finely grate in the Parmesan and whiz until smooth, then pour into a large bowl • Cut the florets off the broccoli, add to the pasta pan and put the lid on

Using a box grater, coarsely grate the broccoli stalk and carrots on to a board • Squeeze and squidge over the avocado, discarding the skin and stone • Roughly chop the tomatoes • Season the salad with salt and pepper, then drizzle with the extra virgin olive oil and balsamic • Add the rocket and toss together

Toast the pine nuts in the frying pan, turning the heat up, and removing when lightly golden • Drain the pasta and broccoli in a colander, reserving a cupful of the starchy cooking water, then tip into the bowl of sauce • Toss together, loosening with a little cooking water, if needed • Pour on to a platter, finely grate over some extra Parmesan, scatter over the toasted pine nuts and serve

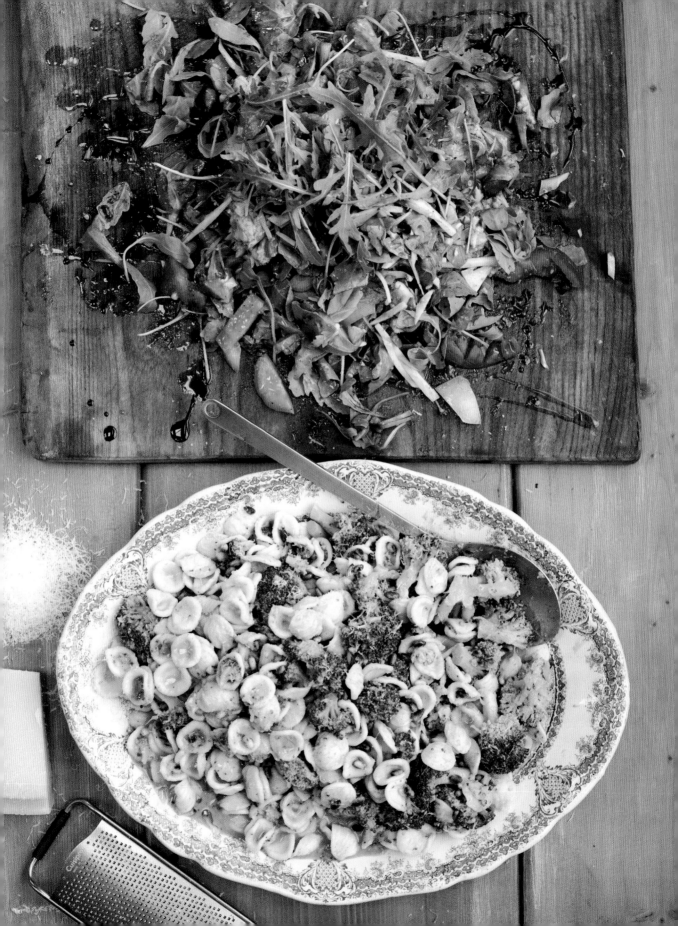

PRAWN LINGUINE
SICILIAN SHAVED FENNEL SALAD

SERVES 4 | 562 CALORIES

Ingredients out • Kettle boiled • Food processor (bowl blade & fine slicer)
• Large non-stick frying pan, medium-high heat • Large lidded pan, medium heat

Breadcrumbs
2 slices of rustic bread (60g)
2 cloves of garlic
extra virgin olive oil

Pasta
320g dried linguine
1 fresh red chilli
4 anchovy fillets
1 good pinch of ground cinnamon
1 pinch of saffron
360g raw peeled tiger prawns
2 cloves of garlic
500g passata
1 lemon
30g Parmesan cheese
a couple of sprigs of fresh basil

Salad
1 bulb of fennel
½ a celery heart
1 bunch of fresh mint
1 lemon

START COOKING

Put the bread and peeled garlic into the processor with 1 tablespoon of oil and blitz into breadcrumbs • Toast these in the large frying pan until golden, tossing regularly • Put the pasta into the large pan, cover with boiling salted water and cook according to packet instructions • Swap to the fine slicer in your processor and slice the halved fennel, trimmed celery, the top leafy half of the mint and the whole lemon • Tip into a serving bowl and toss with 1 tablespoon of oil and a pinch of salt and pepper

Tip the breadcrumbs into a small bowl and put the pan back on a low heat • Finely chop the chilli and put into the frying pan with the anchovies and a little of their oil, the cinnamon, saffron and prawns, then turn up the heat • Squash in the unpeeled garlic through a garlic crusher, add the passata and bring to the boil

Squeeze the lemon juice into the frying pan, then use tongs to transfer the spaghetti straight into the sauce • Finely grate in the Parmesan, toss to coat, then season to taste • Transfer the pasta to a platter, loosening with a splash of cooking water, if needed, pick over the basil leaves and serve with the breadcrumbs and salad on the side

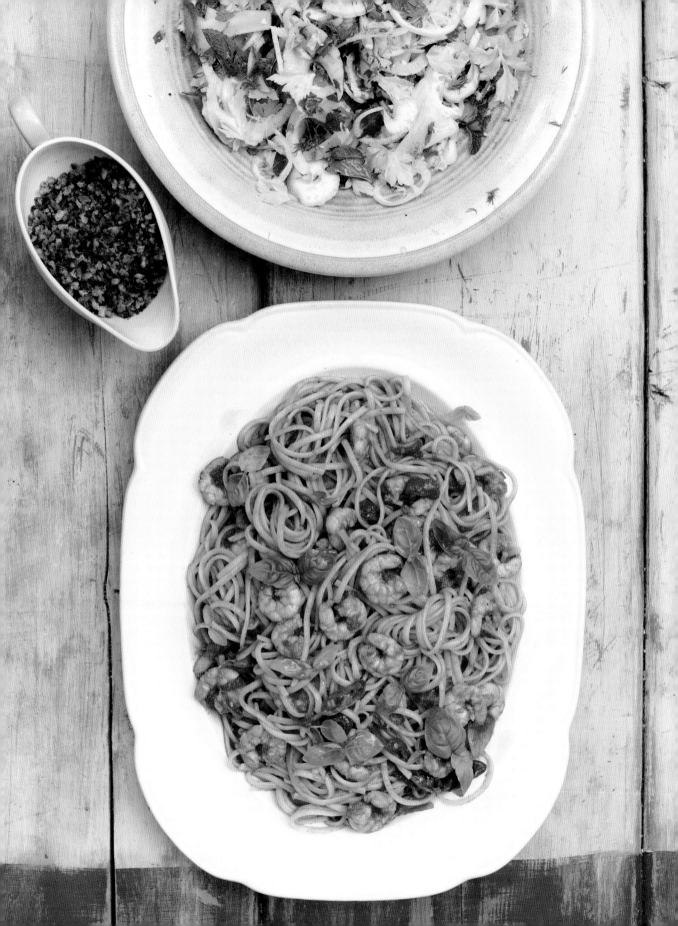

MUSHROOM FARFALLE
BLUE CHEESE, HAZELNUT & APPLE SALAD

SERVES 4 | 586 CALORIES

Ingredients out • *Kettle boiled* • *Large frying pan, medium-high heat* • *Large lidded pan, high heat* • *Small frying pan, medium heat* • *Food processor (bowl blade)*

Pasta

25g dried porcini mushrooms
olive oil
2–4 cloves of garlic
½ a small dried chilli
250g chestnut mushrooms
6 sprigs of fresh thyme
320g dried farfalle
1 tsp truffle oil
1 lemon
½ a bunch of fresh flat-leaf parsley
150g low-fat cottage cheese

Salad

50g blanched hazelnuts
200g baby spinach
1 eating apple
40g blue cheese
1 tsp extra virgin olive oil

START COOKING

Put the porcini into a mug and just cover with boiling water • Put 2 tablespoons of olive oil into the large frying pan, squash in the unpeeled garlic through a garlic crusher, crumble in the dried chilli and tear in the mushrooms • Strip in the thyme leaves, then add the soaked porcini and toss and fry for a few minutes • Put the pasta into the large pan, cover with boiling salted water and cook according to packet instructions

Toast the hazelnuts in the small frying pan until golden, tossing regularly • Put the spinach into a salad bowl, coarsely grate over or matchstick and add the apple, then crumble over the blue cheese • Crush the toasted nuts in a pestle and mortar, then scatter over the salad • Tip the mushrooms into the processor and whiz until fairly smooth, then return to the pan and add 3 small ladles of pasta cooking water and the truffle oil, season to taste and simmer gently

Drain the pasta, reserving a cupful of the starchy cooking water, then toss the pasta with the sauce, loosening with a splash of cooking water, if needed • Finely grate over the lemon zest, finely chop and add most of the top leafy half of the parsley along with the cottage cheese, then toss together and serve straight away • Drizzle the salad with extra virgin olive oil, squeeze over the juice of the zested lemon and serve on the side

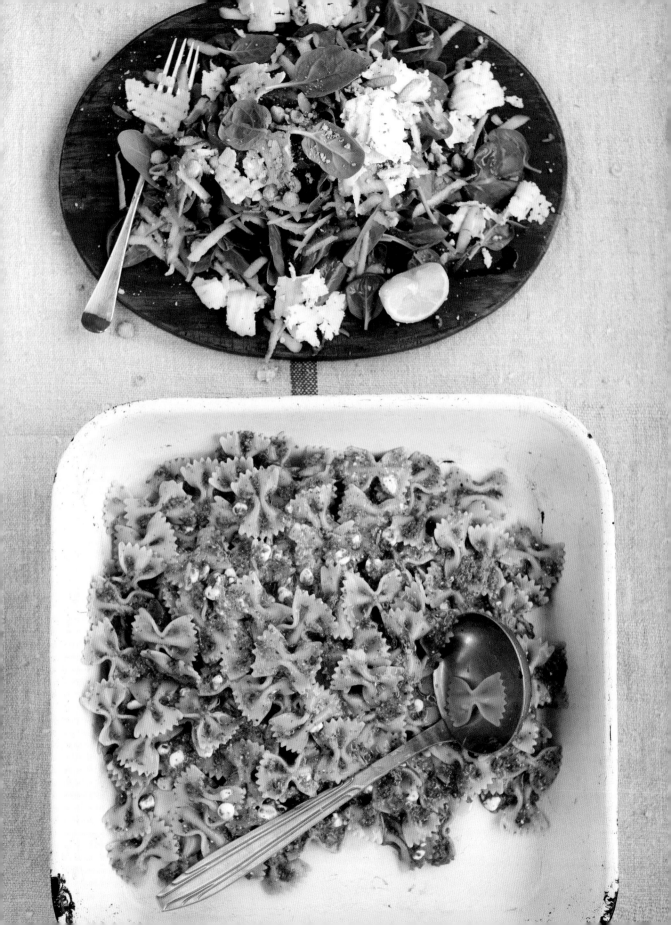

SALSA VERDE TUNA
SICILIAN TOMATO & PASTA SALAD

SERVES 4 | 651 CALORIES

Ingredients out • Kettle boiled • Large lidded pan, high heat
• Food processor (bowl blade) • Large frying pan, medium heat

Pasta & tuna
320g dried pasta shells
8 black olives (stone in)
400g ripe mixed-colour tomatoes
4 jarred red peppers
70g rocket
4 x 120g yellowfin tuna steaks
1 tsp dried oregano
1 tsp fennel seeds
olive oil
1 fresh red chilli
20g Parmesan cheese
1 lemon

Salsa verde
1 big bunch of fresh mint
1 big bunch of fresh flat-leaf parsley
1 lemon
2 anchovy fillets
2 tsp capers (drained)
1 clove of garlic
4 tbsp extra virgin olive oil
1 heaped tsp Dijon mustard
1 tbsp white wine vinegar

START COOKING

Put the pasta into the large pan, cover with boiling salted water and cook according to packet instructions • Rip the top leafy half of the mint and parsley into the processor, squeeze in the lemon juice, add all the other salsa verde ingredients (peel the garlic) and blitz until fine, then season to taste, loosen with 2 tablespoons of water and set aside

Squash the olives (discarding the stones), randomly cut up the tomatoes and peppers, and put them all into a large bowl, then roughly chop and pile the rocket on top • Rub the tuna with salt, pepper, the oregano and fennel seeds, then drizzle with 1 tablespoon of olive oil, put into the frying pan and cook for 1½ minutes on each side, ideally so the tuna's blushing in the middle

Drain the pasta, reserving a cupful of the starchy cooking water, then add to the tomato bowl, toss with half of the salsa verde, loosening with a splash of cooking water, if needed, then pour on to a nice platter • Put the tuna on top, spoon over the remaining salsa verde, scatter with the finely sliced red chilli, then shave over a little Parmesan with a speed-peeler and serve with lemon wedges

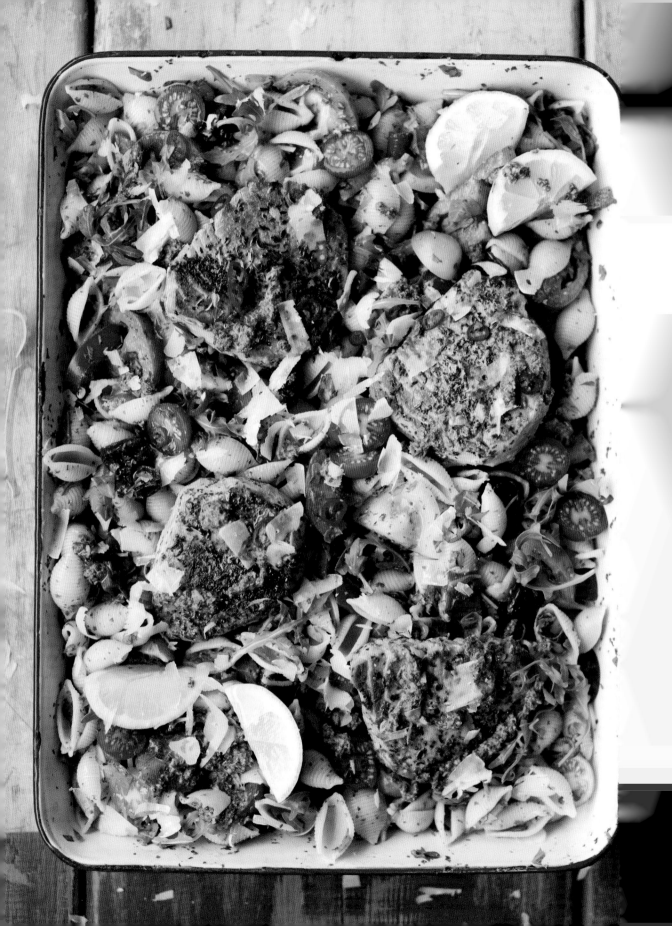

PESTO SPAGHETTI
LEMON-STEAMED FISH

SERVES 4 | 649 CALORIES

Ingredients out • Kettle boiled • Wok or large pan, medium heat • Large lidded pan, medium heat • Food processor (bowl blade) • Two 25cm bamboo steamers

Fish

200g large scallops
400g white fish fillets,
  scaled and pin-boned
olive oil
1 lemon
½ a dried red chilli

Pasta

320g dried spaghetti
200g green beans
200g purple sprouting broccoli

Pesto

75g blanched almonds
1 big bunch of fresh basil
1 clove of garlic
2 tbsp extra virgin olive oil
50g Parmesan cheese
1 lemon

START COOKING

Score the scallops on one side in deep crisscrosses • Pour 2.5cm of boiling water into the wok or large pan • Pour the rest of the water into the other pan, add the spaghetti and a pinch of salt and cook according to packet instructions • Put the almonds into the processor, rip in most of the basil leaves and squash in the unpeeled garlic through a garlic crusher • Add the extra virgin olive oil, Parmesan and the juice from ½ a lemon, blitz until smooth, then season to taste and check the balance of flavours – it should be clean and refreshing

Line the beans up and cut off the stalks, then add to the pasta pan • Put one of the steamers into the wok and add the trimmed broccoli, then put the second steamer on top • Rub the fish and scallops with a pinch of salt and pepper and lay in the second steamer • Drizzle with 1 tablespoon of olive oil, finely grate over the zest of a lemon and squeeze over half the juice, then crumble over the chilli and put the steamer lid on until cooked through

Drain the pasta and beans, reserving a cupful of the starchy cooking water, then return them to the pan • Spoon in the pesto from the processor and toss together, loosening with splashes of the cooking water until silky • Squeeze in lemon juice to taste, then pour into a serving bowl with the broccoli • Sprinkle over the remaining basil leaves and serve alongside the steamer basket of fish

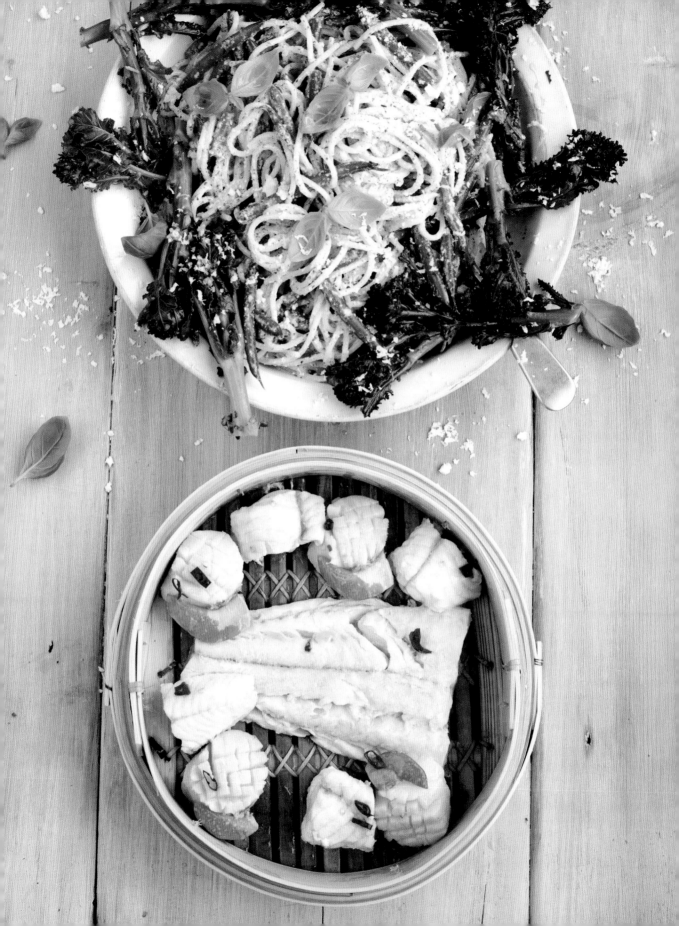

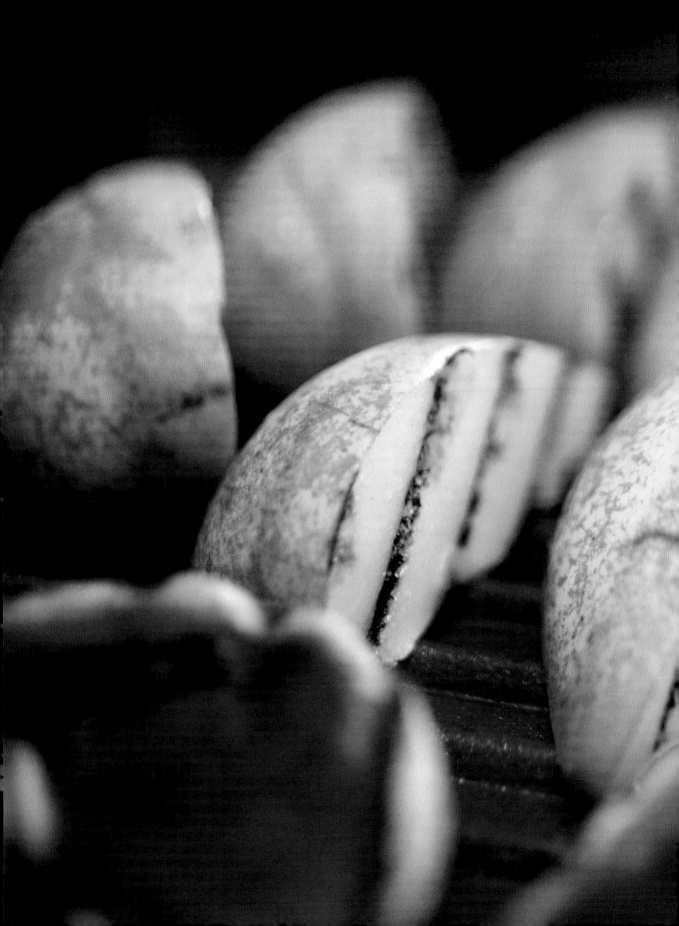

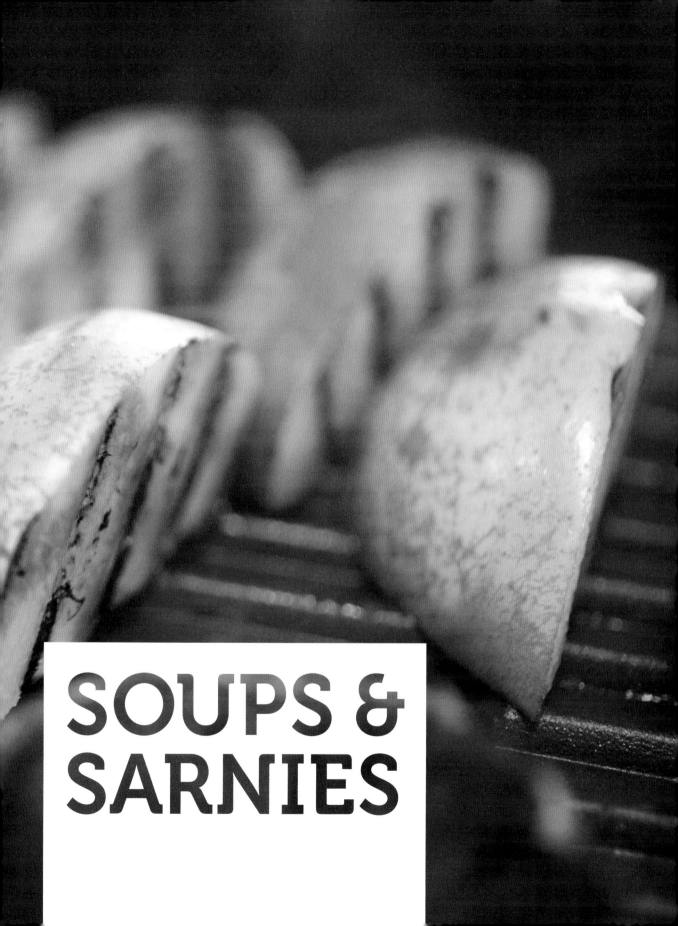

SOUPS & SARNIES

MEXICAN TOMATO SOUP
CHILLI NACHOS, VEGGIE & FETA SPRINKLES

Ingredients out • Kettle boiled • Oven grill on high
• Large lidded pan, high heat • Stick blender

Soup

1 small bunch of spring onions
olive oil
1 bunch of fresh coriander
4 cloves of garlic
100g basmati rice
450g jarred red peppers
2 x 400g tins of chopped tomatoes
250ml fat-free natural yoghurt
2 tsp pickled jalapeño chillies
½ a bunch of fresh mint
2 limes

Sprinkles

1 handful of cherry tomatoes
1 ripe avocado
30g feta cheese

Nachos

2–3 fresh red and green chillies
175g low-salt tortilla chips
50g Cheddar cheese

START COOKING

Trim and finely slice the spring onions (reserving some for garnish) and put into the pan with 2 tablespoons of oil • Tear in the coriander stalks (reserving the leaves) • Squash in the unpeeled garlic through a garlic crusher and add the rice, drained jarred peppers, and the tinned tomatoes • Pour in 850ml of boiling water, add a pinch of salt and cover with the lid

Quarter the cherry tomatoes, halve the avocado (discarding the stone) and place on a serving board with the reserved spring onions and coriander leaves, and the feta • Finely slice the chillies and add half to the board • Empty the tortilla chips on to a baking tray, grate over the Cheddar and scatter over the remaining chillies, then pop under the grill on the top shelf until the cheese is melted, removing when golden

In a bowl, use the stick blender to blitz the yoghurt and jalapeño chillies with a splash of their pickling vinegar and the top leafy half of the mint until nice and smooth • Next use the stick blender to blitz the soup until smooth, add the juice of ½ a lime, season well to taste, then either enjoy it thick, or add some water to thin it down • Drizzle over the spiked yoghurt, and serve with the nachos, sprinkles and lime wedges

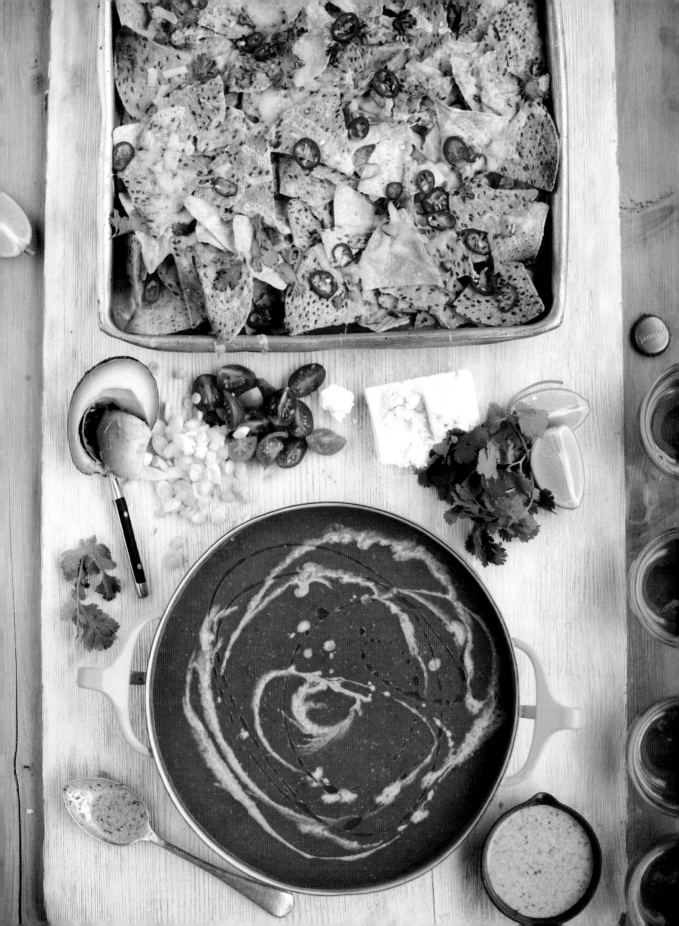

MINESTRONE
POACHED CHICKEN & SALSA VERDE

SERVES 4 | 608 CALORIES

Ingredients out • Kettle boiled • Large lidded casserole pan, medium heat • Food processor (thick slicer & bowl blade)

Chicken & soup
6 rashers of smoked pancetta
olive oil
2 sprigs of fresh rosemary
2 small carrots
2 sticks of celery
1 red onion
2 chicken stock cubes
½ a head of broccoli
½ a cauliflower
100g basmati rice
100g dried macaroni
2 x 150g skinless chicken breasts
1 handful of frozen broad beans
1 handful of frozen peas
200g baby spinach
Parmesan cheese, to serve

Salsa verde
1 bunch of fresh tarragon
  or flat-leaf parsley
1 bunch of fresh mint
2 anchovy fillets
1 tbsp cornichons
1 tbsp capers
1 heaped tsp Dijon mustard
1 clove of garlic
3 tbsp extra virgin olive oil
1 tbsp cider vinegar

START COOKING

Finely slice the pancetta and put it into the casserole pan with 2 tablespoons of olive oil, strip in the rosemary leaves and cook until crispy, then remove it all to a bowl, leaving the oil behind • Take the pan off the heat • Slice the trimmed carrots and celery and peeled onion in the processor then tip into the pan • Put back on a high heat, add salt, pepper and crumble in the stock cubes • Slice the broccoli stalks (reserving the florets) and all of the cauliflower in the processor and tip into the pan along with the rice and macaroni, then cover with 1.5 litres of boiling water and the lid

On a plastic board, bash the fatter end of the chicken breasts with a rolling pin so they're an even thickness, then add to the pan, making sure they're fully submerged, and cover with the lid • Swap to the bowl blade in the processor • Put the tarragon or parsley, the top leafy half of the mint, the anchovies, cornichons, capers and mustard in the processor • Squash in the unpeeled garlic through a garlic crusher and blitz until fine • Scrape into a bowl, add 1 tablespoon of the soup stock, the extra virgin olive oil and vinegar and mix together, loosening with an extra splash of stock, if needed

After about 8 minutes, scoop out the cooked chicken, then add the broccoli florets, broad beans, peas and spinach to the soup, replacing the lid • Spoon the salsa verde on to a platter, slice the chicken breasts, then serve them on top of the salsa, sprinkled with the crispy pancetta and rosemary • Add more boiling water to the soup if you prefer it brothy, then serve with a few shavings of Parmesan, mixing everything together at the table

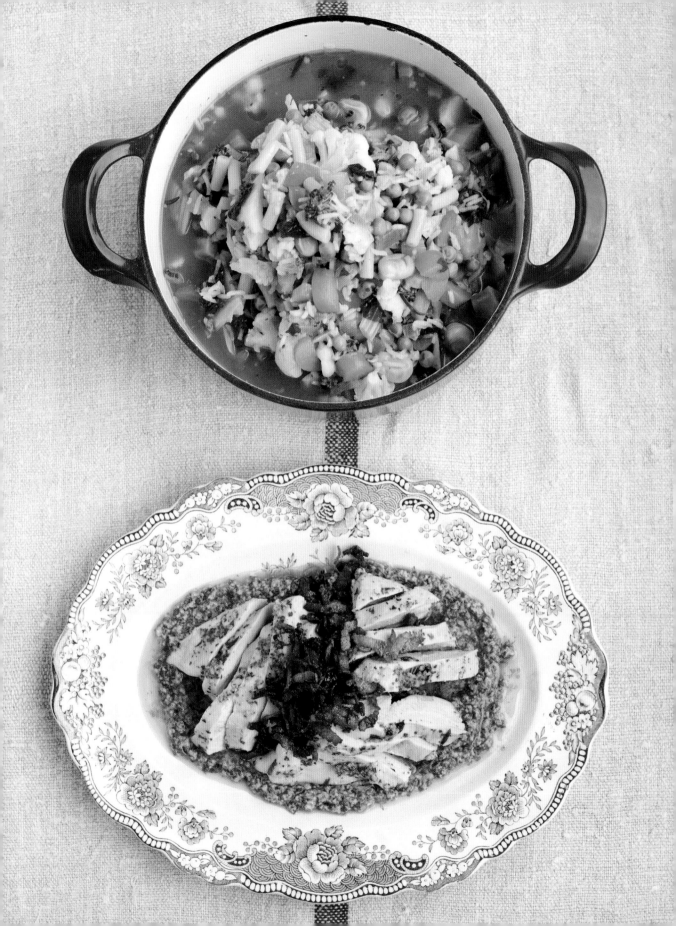

MUSHROOM SOUP
STILTON, APPLE & WALNUT CROÛTES

SERVES 4 | 405 CALORIES

Ingredients out • Kettle boiled • Oven grill on high • Large lidded pan, medium heat • Griddle pan, high heat • Stick blender

Soup

2 onions
olive oil
1 chicken or vegetable stock cube
½ a bunch of fresh thyme
2 cloves of garlic
4 large portobello mushrooms
100g basmati rice
1 tbsp single cream
1 tsp truffle oil

Croûtes

8 chestnut mushrooms
1 ciabatta loaf
1 clove of garlic
1 eating apple
½ a bunch of fresh
  curly parsley
1 lemon
50g Stilton cheese
1 small handful of shelled walnuts

START COOKING

Peel, halve and finely slice the onions and put them into the large pan with 2 tablespoons of olive oil • Crumble in the stock cube, add a pinch of salt and pepper, strip in the thyme leaves and squash in 2 unpeeled cloves of garlic through a garlic crusher • De-stalk the chestnut mushrooms and place the tops on the griddle pan, turning when charred • Tear the chestnut stalks and portobellos into the onion pan, add the rice and cook for a couple of minutes • Pour in 1 litre of boiling water and boil with the lid on

Cut 4 slices of ciabatta at an angle and add to the griddle pan • When charred on both sides, rub with a halved garlic clove • Coarsely grate or slice the apple into matchsticks and toss with the roughly chopped parsley and a little lemon juice • Place the chestnut mushrooms on the toasts, crumble over the stilton and walnuts, then pop under the grill until the cheese is melted

Use the stick blender to purée the soup to a consistency you like, then season to taste, if needed, and swirl in the cream and truffle oil • Top the toasts with pinches of apple and parsley and serve on the side

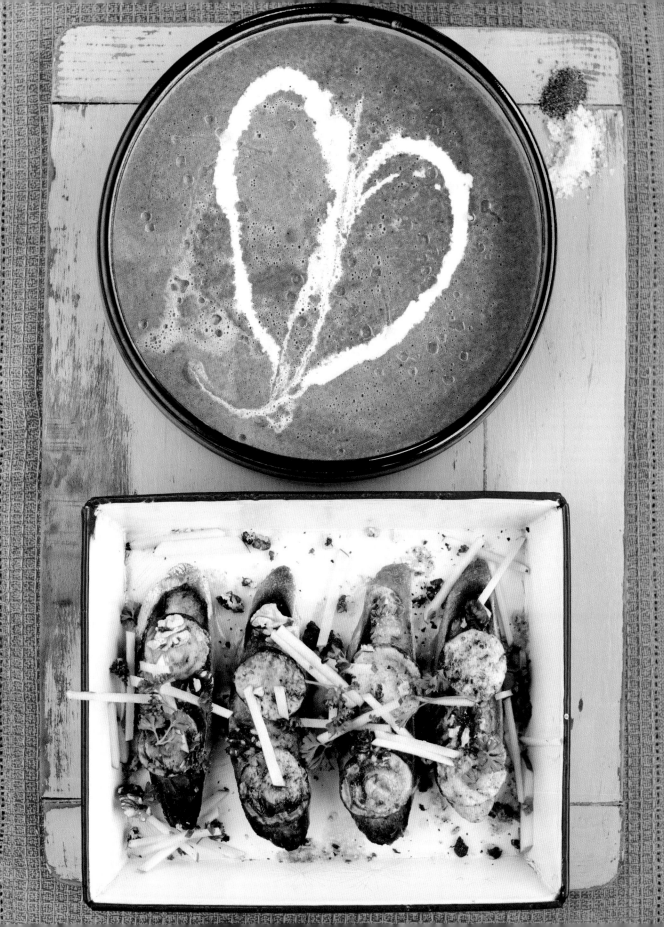

SQUASH SOUP
SAGEY CHESTNUT DUMPLINGS

SERVES 4 | 484 CALORIES

Ingredients out • Kettle boiled • Food processor (bowl blade) • Large lidded casserole pan, medium heat • Large lidded pan, high heat • Stick blender

Soup

1 bunch of spring onions
a few sprigs of fresh rosemary
1 fresh red chilli
1 chicken stock cube
olive oil
1 medium butternut squash
   (neck end only)
3 carrots
1 x 400g tin of chickpeas

Dumplings

100g vac-packed chestnuts
100g self-raising flour,
   plus extra for dusting
1 chicken stock cube
8 rashers of smoked pancetta
10 fresh sage leaves
1 whole nutmeg, for grating
optional: 30g Cheddar cheese

START COOKING

Trim the spring onions and blitz in the processor with the rosemary leaves, chilli and stock cube until fine, then put into the casserole pan with 1 tablespoon of oil • Cut the neck off the squash, trimming away the stalky end, then carefully quarter (don't peel, and keep the seed end for another day) • Blitz the squash in the processor with the trimmed carrots until finely chopped • Add to the casserole pan with the chickpeas, their water, and 1 litre of boiling water • Cover with the lid and cook on high • Refill and boil the kettle

Blitz the chestnuts, flour, stock cube and a pinch of pepper in the processor • Start adding 100ml of cold water, a splash at a time, until it just comes together as a ball of firm dough • Split the dough in half and roll each piece into a sausage shape on a flour-dusted surface, then cut into 2cm chunks • Fill the large pan with boiling water, add the dumplings, cover with the lid and simmer on a medium heat for 6 minutes, or until fluffy

Blitz the soup with the stick blender until lovely and smooth, then season to taste and simmer until ready to serve • Put the pancetta into a deep roasting tray on a high heat with 1 tablespoon of oil • When it starts to crisp up, add the sage leaves • Scoop out the fluffy dumplings with a slotted spoon, toss in the tray of crispy pancetta and sage, then finely grate over half the nutmeg and serve with a grating of Cheddar, if you like

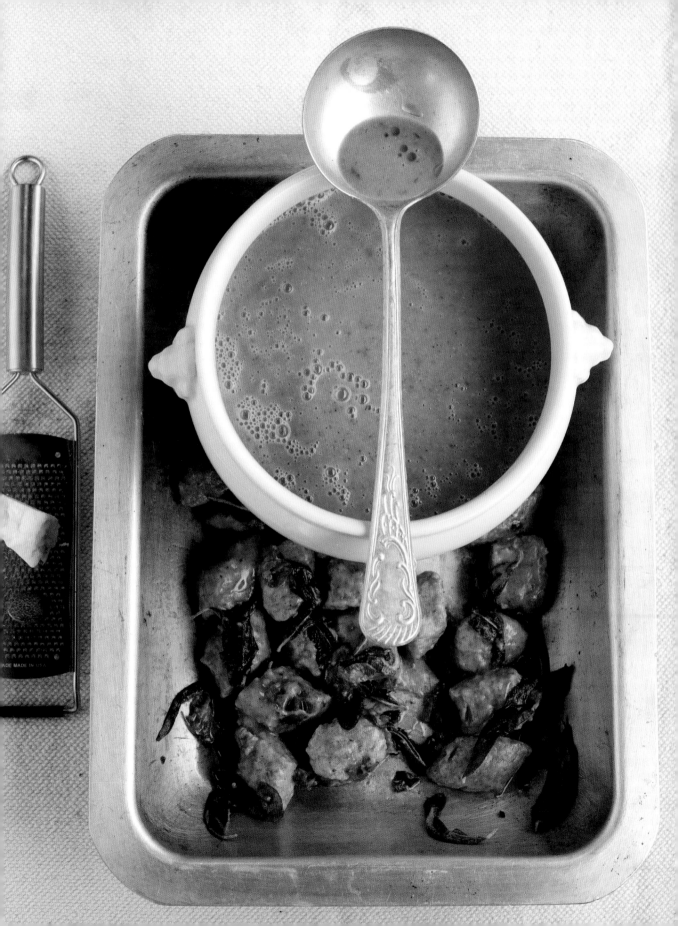

MEXICAN BLT
CHILLIES, GUACAMOLE & SALAD

SERVES 4 | 638 CALORIES

Ingredients out • Oven at 130°C/250°F/gas ½
• Medium frying pan, medium-high heat • Food processor (bowl blade)

BLT
4 rashers of smoked pancetta
2 x 180g skinless chicken breasts
1 pinch of dried oregano
1 pinch of cumin seeds
1 baguette

Salad
1 little gem lettuce
1 bunch of radishes
2 punnets of cress
40g feta cheese
2 tbsp red wine vinegar
2 tbsp extra virgin olive oil
8 pickled green chillies

Guacamole
½ a bunch of fresh coriander
1 fresh red chilli
4 spring onions
2 ripe avocados
5 ripe cherry tomatoes
2 limes

START COOKING

Put the pancetta into the frying pan, removing when golden • On a large sheet of greaseproof paper, toss the chicken with salt, pepper, the oregano and cumin • Fold over the paper and bash and flatten the chicken to about 1.5cm thick with a rolling pin • Add the chicken to the pan, turning after 3 to 4 minutes, until golden and cooked through • Pop the baguette into the oven • Cut the lettuce into wedges, halve the radishes and pile on a board, then snip over the cress and crumble over the feta

Mix the vinegar, extra virgin olive oil and a pinch of salt and pepper in a small bowl and pop on the board with a pile of pickled chillies • In the processor, pulse most of the coriander, the chilli and trimmed spring onions until fairly fine • Squash out and add the avocado flesh (discarding the skin and stones) along with the tomatoes, then squeeze in the juice from 1½ limes, pulse again, and season to taste

Return the crispy pancetta to the chicken pan to warm through • Get the bread out of the oven and cut it in half lengthways • Spoon the guacamole over the bread, tear over one of the lettuce wedges, slice up and add the chicken and pancetta and drizzle over any pan juices, then scatter with the remaining coriander leaves • Serve with lime wedges, pickled chillies and the salad, dressing it at the table

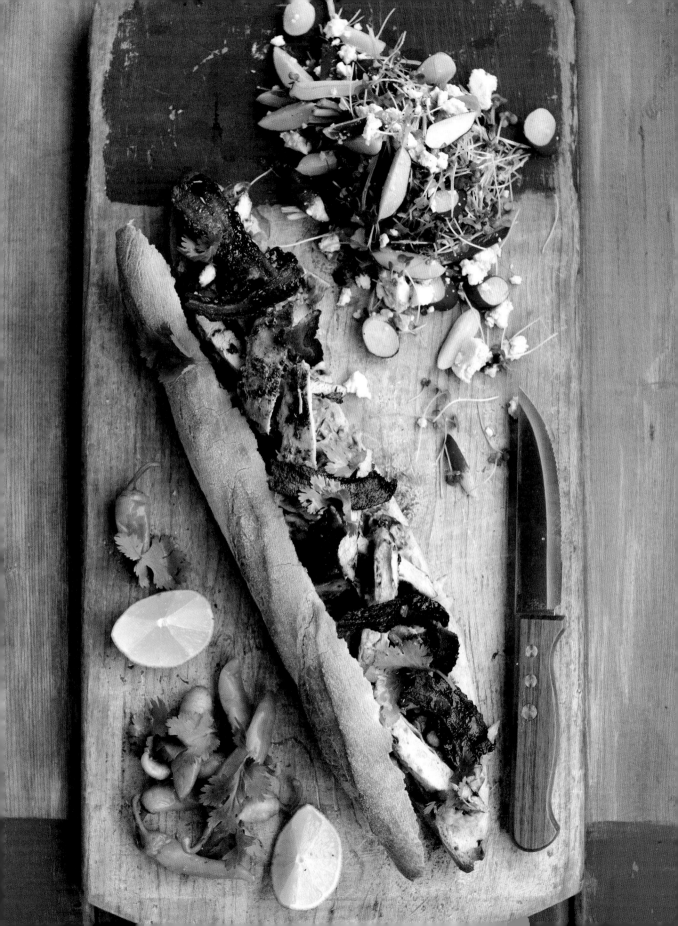

THE BEST FISH BAPS
MUSHY PEAS & TARTARE SAUCE

SERVES 4 | 665 CALORIES

Ingredients out • Kettle boiled • Oven at 130°C/250°F/gas ½ • Small lidded pan, high heat • Large frying pan, high heat • Food processor (bowl blade)

Baps

4 nice soft wholewheat baps

4 large (halved) or 8 small flat-fish
fillets (roughly 480g in total),
such as plaice, lemon sole,
megrim or dab, skin off and
pin-boned

1 pinch of cayenne pepper

½ a mug of plain flour

olive oil

25g Parmesan cheese

1 punnet of cress

1 lemon

Peas

1 medium potato

500g frozen peas

½ a bunch of fresh mint

Sauce

6 cornichons

1 tbsp capers

1 little gem lettuce

250g fat-free natural yoghurt

¼ of a bunch of fresh
flat-leaf parsley

1 lemon

START COOKING

Put the baps into the oven • Slice the potato 0.5cm thick, put it into the small pan, cover with boiling water and the lid and bring to the boil • On a sheet of greaseproof paper, season the fish with salt, pepper and the cayenne, then sprinkle over the flour to coat

Pour 2 tablespoons of oil into the frying pan and add the fish • Cook until golden, finely grating the Parmesan over the top when you flip it over • Tip the frozen peas into the pan with the potato, then rip in the leafy top half of the mint and replace the lid

Put the cornichons, capers, lettuce and yoghurt into the processor • Tear in the top leafy half of the parsley, squeeze in the lemon juice, then whiz up, season to taste and pour into a bowl • Drain the peas and potatoes, purée in the processor and season to taste • When the fish is perfect, get the baps out of the oven and serve with the peas, tartare sauce, pinches of cress and lemon wedges

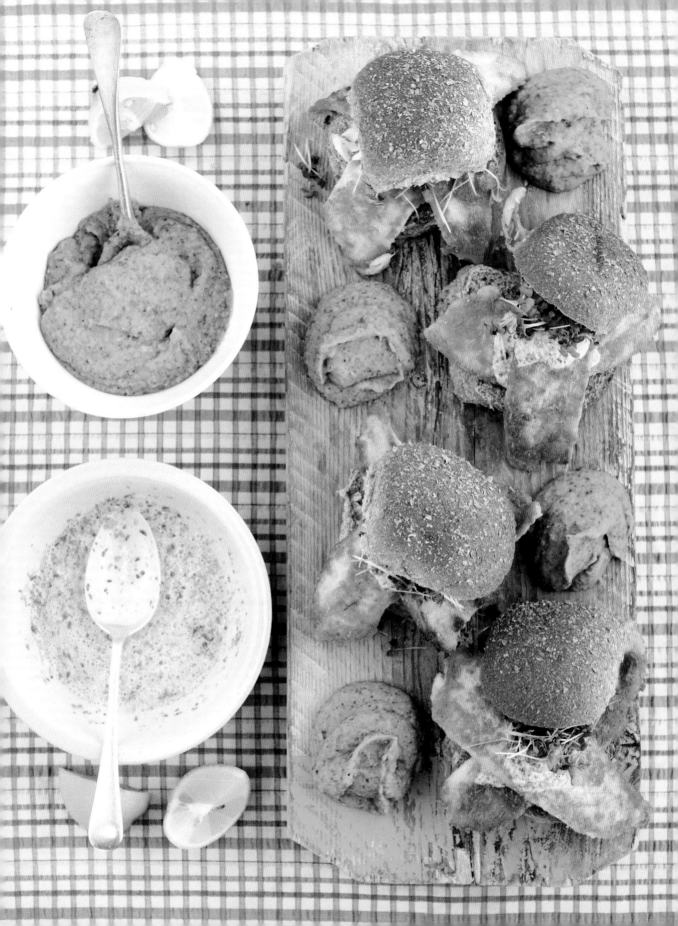

GRILLED MUSHROOM SUB
SMOKY PANCETTA, MELTED CHEESE & PEARS

SERVES 4 | 491 CALORIES

Ingredients out • Oven grill on high • Griddle pan, high heat

Sub

1 ciabatta loaf
4 large portobello mushrooms
50g Emmental cheese
½ a bunch of fresh thyme
½ a clove of garlic
2 ripe pears
8 rashers of smoked pancetta
1 tsp runny honey
2 large ripe tomatoes
125g low-fat cottage cheese
½ a lemon

Salad

1 round lettuce
1 red chicory
100g watercress
1 bunch of radishes
1 handful of shelled walnuts
5 cornichons
1 tbsp white wine vinegar
2 tbsp extra virgin olive oil
1 tsp Dijon mustard

START COOKING

Place the ciabatta at the bottom of the grill • Cut off and discard the mushroom stalks, then lay the tops on the griddle pan • Quarter the lettuce, finely slice the base of the chicory and click the upper leaves apart, then put both in a large bowl with the watercress and halved radishes • Crumble over the walnuts, then chop and add the cornichons

In a separate bowl, mix the vinegar with the oil, mustard, salt and pepper • Transfer the mushrooms to a roasting tray, then slice and lay over the Emmental • Pick over the thyme leaves, squash over the unpeeled garlic through a garlic crusher and pop under the grill until the cheese is melted

Quarter the pears and put on the griddle pan, turning when golden and adding the pancetta to the pan to crisp up at the same time, then drizzle the honey over the pears for the last 30 seconds • Slice the tomatoes • In a bowl, mix the cottage cheese with the zest and juice of ½ a lemon and a pinch of salt and pepper • Slice open the hot ciabatta and load it up with all your fillings • Dress the salad at the last minute and serve

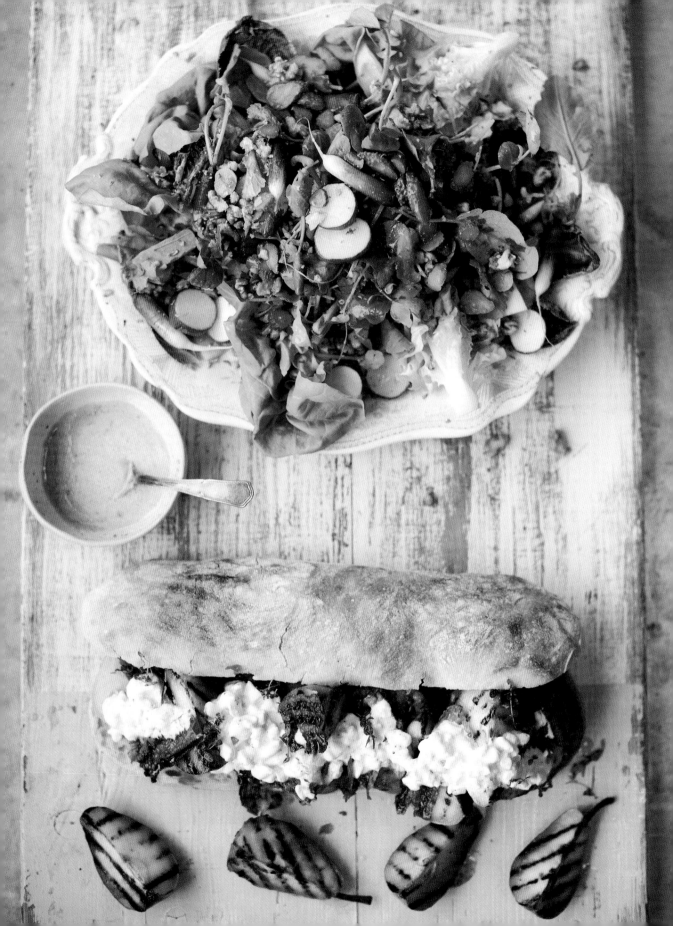

TAPAS BRUSCHETTA
GOLDEN GRILLED SARDINES

Ingredients out • Oven at 200°C/400°F/gas 6 • Food processor (fine slicer & bowl blade) • Griddle pan, high heat

Bruschetta

2 ciabatta loaves
250g cooked vac-packed beetroot
balsamic vinegar
1 bunch of fresh basil
1 small bulb of fennel
1 lemon
a few sprigs of fresh mint
1 clove of garlic
8 ripe cherry tomatoes
4 rashers of prosciutto

Sardines

8 x 80g whole sardines,
   scaled and gutted
1 pinch of cayenne pepper

Houmous

1 x 400g tin of chickpeas
1 heaped tsp smooth peanut butter
1 lemon
1 pinch of cumin seeds
2–3 tbsp fat-free
   natural yoghurt

START COOKING

Trim the edges off the ciabatta lengthways, then cut them in half lengthways and put into the oven to toast, removing when golden • Tip the beetroot into a shallow bowl, then mash with a potato masher • Drizzle with a little balsamic and season with salt and pepper • Roughly chop half of the basil leaves and toss with the beetroot

Quarter the fennel bulb, then finely slice it in the processor along with ½ a lemon • Chop the top leafy half off the mint, then add to the bowl, toss together and season to taste • Lightly season the sardines with salt, pepper and the cayenne, then place on the griddle to cook for around 3 minutes on each side, or until golden

Swap to the standard blade in the processor • Add the drained chickpeas, peanut butter and the juice of 1 lemon • Rip off and add the remaining basil leaves, cumin seeds and yoghurt, then whiz until smooth and season to taste • Rub the toasts with half a garlic clove and the tomatoes, then lay them on a nice serving board with the prosciutto • Squeeze lemon juice over the sardines, then take everything to the table and load up the toasts however you like them

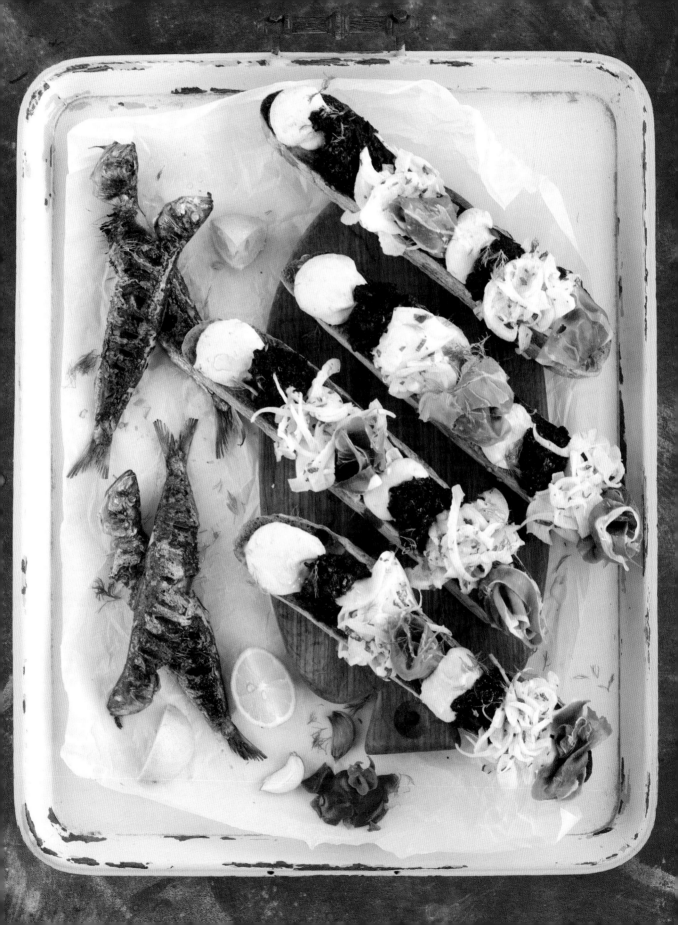

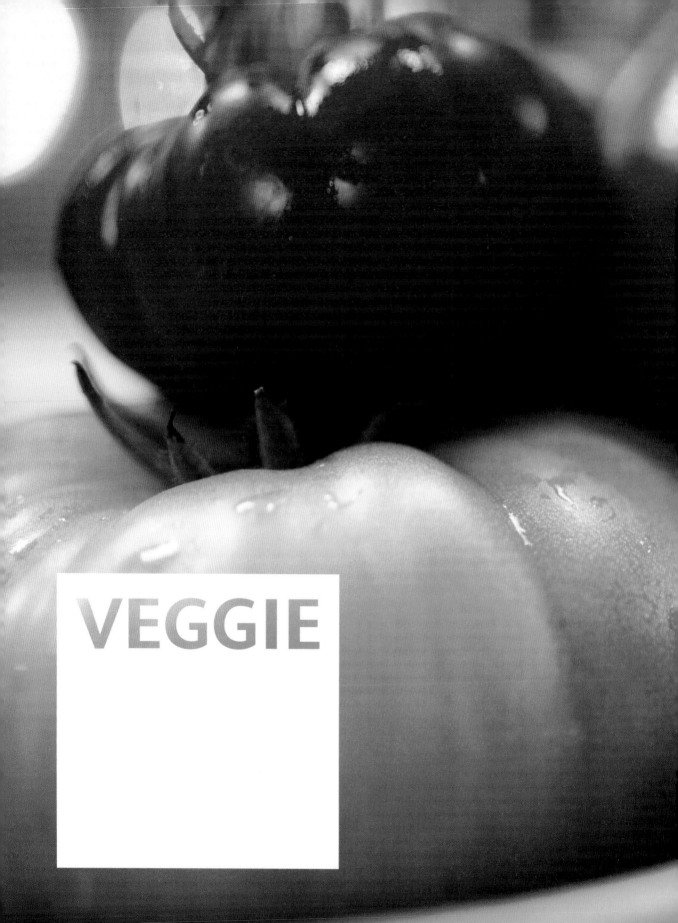

VEGGIE

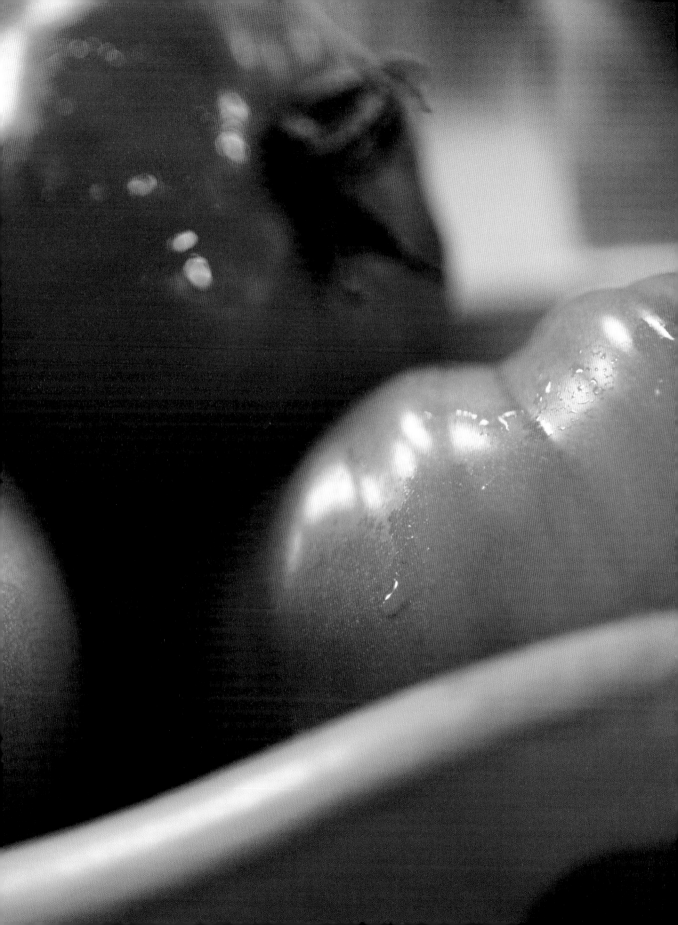

HAPPY COW BURGERS
OLD-SCHOOL COLESLAW & CORN ON THE COB

SERVES 4 | 619 CALORIES

Ingredients out ∘ Kettle boiled ∘ Oven at 130°C/250°F/gas ½ ∘ Large lidded pan, medium heat ∘ Food processor (bowl blade & coarse grater) ∘ Large frying pan, medium-high heat

Corn

4 corn on the cob
1 tsp extra virgin olive oil
1 lime
1 pinch of cayenne pepper

Burgers

1 big bunch of fresh coriander
1 x 400g tin of mixed beans
200g frozen broad beans
½ tsp cayenne pepper
½ tsp ground cumin
½ tsp ground coriander
1 lemon
1 heaped tbsp plain flour,
   plus extra for dusting
olive oil
2 large ripe tomatoes
1 little gem lettuce
4 gherkins
75g feta cheese
4 burger baps
tomato ketchup, to serve

Slaw

½ a small white and red cabbage
   (roughly 200g of each)
½ a red onion
4 heaped tbsp fat-free
   natural yoghurt
1 heaped tsp wholegrain mustard

START COOKING

Put the corn into the pan and cover with boiling water and the lid ∘ Put the coriander stalks into the processor (reserving the leaves), then drain the mixed beans and add, along with the broad beans, a pinch of salt and pepper, the cayenne, cumin, ground coriander, grated lemon zest and flour ∘ Whiz until fine and combined, scraping down the sides of the processor if needed

Tip the mixture on to a generously flour-dusted board, divide into 4 pieces, then roll each piece into a ball and flatten into a patty about 2.5cm thick, dusting your hands and the burgers with flour as you go ∘ Pour 2 tablespoons of olive oil into the frying pan, followed by the burgers, pressing them down with a fish slice and flipping them when golden ∘ Slice the tomatoes, lettuce and gherkins on a nice serving board and crumble the feta on one side ∘ Put the baps into the oven

Swap to the grater in the processor, then grate the cabbages and peeled red onion, and tip into a bowl ∘ Chop the coriander leaves and add, with the yoghurt, mustard and the juice of the zested lemon, then toss well and season to taste ∘ Drain the corn, place on a platter, drizzle with the extra virgin olive oil and lime juice, and sprinkle with a pinch of salt and the cayenne ∘ Get the buns out of the oven, cut them in half, dollop with ketchup, add the burgers and let everyone build their own

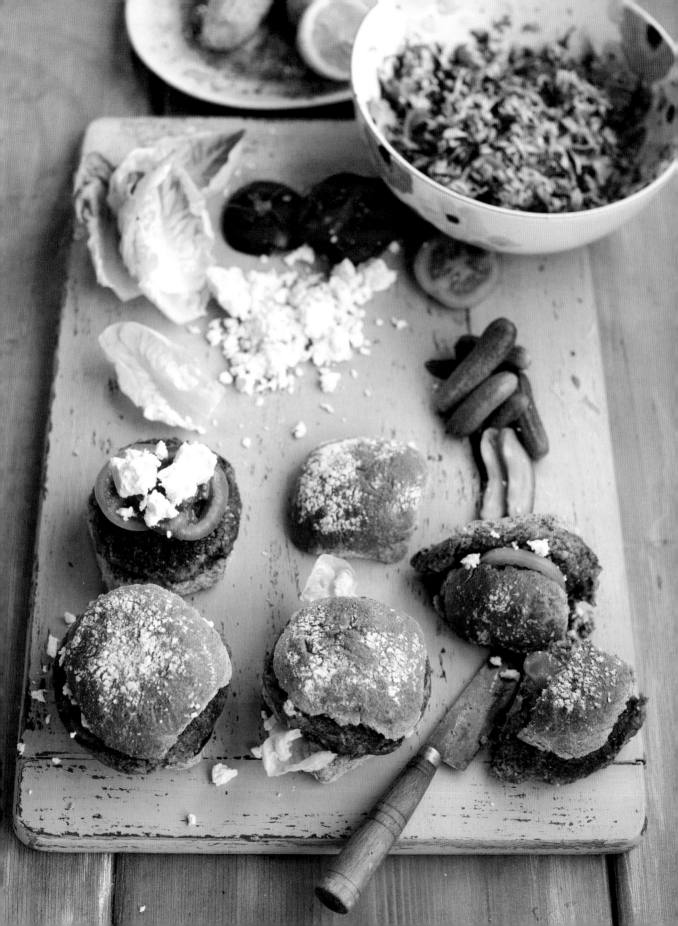

VEGGIE CHILLI
CRUNCHY TORTILLA & AVOCADO SALAD

SERVES 4 | 749 CALORIES

Ingredients out • Oven at 200°C/400°F/gas 6 • Food processor (bowl blade)
• Lidded casserole pan, high heat • Stick blender

Chilli & rice

1 dried smoked chipotle
  or ancho chilli
½ a fresh red chilli
1 red onion
1 tsp sweet smoked paprika
½ tsp cumin seeds
1–2 garlic cloves
1 big bunch of fresh coriander
olive oil
2 mixed-colour peppers
1 x 400g tin of chickpeas
1 x 400g tin of black beans
700g passata
1x 250g pack of cooked
  mixed long grain and wild rice

Salad

4 small corn tortilla wraps
2 ripe avocados
3 heaped tbsp fat-free natural
  yoghurt, plus extra to serve
2 limes
1 romaine lettuce
½ a cucumber
1 fresh red chilli
1 handful of ripe cherry tomatoes

START COOKING

Put the chillies, peeled and halved red onion, paprika and cumin seeds into the processor, squash in the unpeeled garlic through a garlic crusher, then add the coriander stalks (reserving the leaves) and 2 tablespoons of oil, and whiz until fine • Tip into the pan, then add the deseeded and roughly chopped peppers, drained chickpeas and black beans, a pinch of salt and pepper and the passata, stir well and put the lid on • Fold the tortillas in half, slice into 0.5cm strips, sprinkle on to a baking tray and pop in the oven until golden and crisp

Put most of the coriander leaves, a pinch of salt and pepper, half a peeled avocado, the yoghurt and the juice from 2 limes into a jug and whiz with a stick blender until silky • Check and adjust the seasoning of the chilli, leave the lid off • Remove the tortillas from the oven into a bowl, cut the lettuce into chunky wedges and add to the bowl • Scoop and dot over curls of avocado • Peel the cucumber into ribbons and finely slice half a chilli, then scatter both over the top

Make a well in the middle of the chilli and tip in the rice, then pop the lid on for the last few minutes to warm the rice through • Pour the dressing over the salad, pick over the remaining coriander leaves, finely slice the remaining chilli and sprinkle over the top along with the halved cherry tomatoes, then toss everything together • Serve with dollops of yoghurt

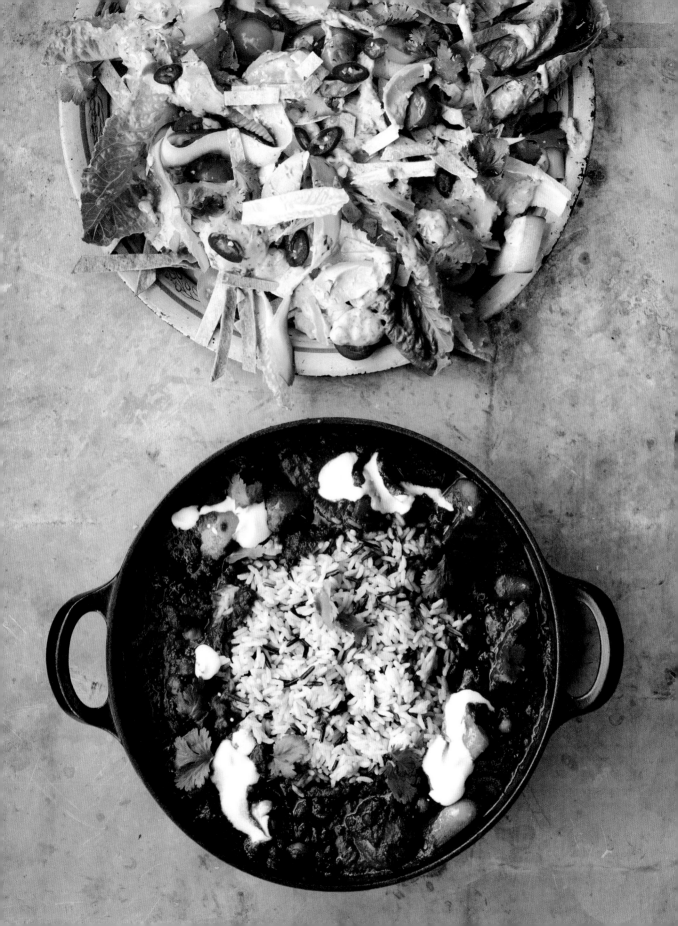

FALAFEL WRAPS
GRILLED VEG & SALSA

SERVES 4 | 602 CALORIES

Ingredients out • Food processor (bowl blade) • Large frying pan, medium heat • Griddle pan, high heat

Falafel
1 x 400g tin of mixed beans
1 x 400g tin of chickpeas
1 lemon
1 tbsp harissa
1 heaped tsp allspice
1 heaped tbsp plain flour
1 bunch of fresh coriander
olive oil

Sides
2 mixed-colour peppers
4 spring onions
8 small wholewheat tortillas
1 tbsp Lingham's chilli sauce
250g low-fat cottage cheese
optional: pickled red cabbage

Salsa
1 big handful of mixed-colour
   ripe tomatoes
½–1 fresh red chilli
½ a clove of garlic
1 lime

START COOKING

Drain the beans and chickpeas and put them into the processor • Finely grate in the lemon zest, then add a pinch of salt and pepper, the harissa, allspice, flour and coriander stalks (reserving the leaves) • Blitz until smooth, scraping down the sides of the processor if needed • Scrape out the mixture and use clean, wet hands to quickly divide and shape it into 8 patties about 1.5cm thick • Put 1 tablespoon of oil into the frying pan and add the falafels, turning when golden and crisp

Rip the seeds and stalks out of the peppers, tear each one into bite-sized chunks and put on the griddle pan with the trimmed and halved spring onions and a pinch of salt and pepper, turning when charred • Put the tomatoes, chilli and half the coriander leaves into the processor • Squash in the unpeeled garlic through a garlic crusher, squeeze in the lime juice, whiz until fine, then season to taste and pour into a serving dish

Pop the tortillas into the microwave (800W) for 45 seconds while you marble the chilli sauce into the cottage cheese • Squeeze the juice of half the zested lemon over the charred veggies, then take with the falafels to the table, scattering everything with the rest of the coriander • Let everyone assemble their own wraps, and serve with pickled red cabbage, if you like

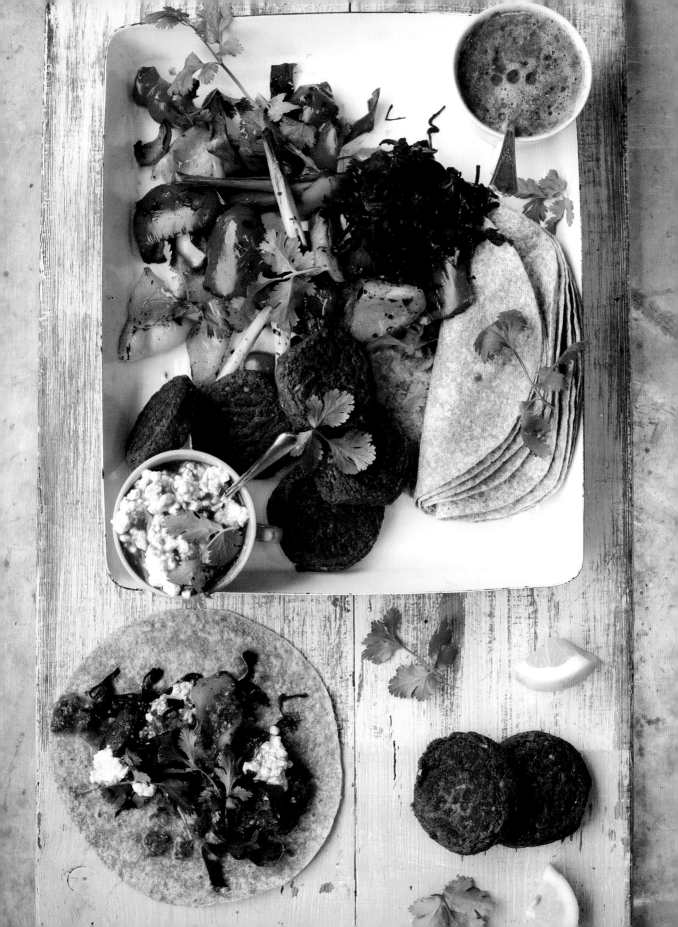

KERALAN VEGGIE CURRY
POPPADOMS, RICE & MINTY YOGHURT

SERVES 4 | 725 CALORIES

Ingredients out • Kettle boiled • Griddle pan, high heat • Medium lidded pan, medium heat • Large casserole pan, low heat • Food processor (bowl blade)

Curry
½ a cauliflower
2 tbsp rapeseed oil
1 heaped tsp black mustard seeds
1 heaped tsp fenugreek seeds
1 heaped tsp turmeric
1 small handful of dried curry
    leaves
1 thumb-sized piece of ginger
2 cloves of garlic
6 spring onions
1 fresh red chilli
1 large bunch of fresh coriander
2 ripe tomatoes
1 x 400g tin of light coconut milk
1 x 400g tin of chickpeas
1 x 227g tin of pineapple chunks
    in juice
1 lemon

Rice
1 mug (300g) of 10-minute
    wholegrain or basmati rice
10 cloves
½ a lemon

To serve
4 uncooked poppadoms
½ a bunch of fresh mint
3 tbsp fat-free natural yoghurt
½ a lemon

START COOKING

Remove the outer leaves from the cauliflower, then slice it 1cm thick and put it on the griddle pan, turning when lightly charred • Put 1 mug of rice and 2 mugs of boiling water into the medium pan with the cloves, lemon half and a pinch of salt, and put the lid on • Pour the oil into the casserole pan, then quickly stir in the mustard and fenugreek seeds, turmeric and curry leaves

Pulse the peeled ginger and garlic, trimmed spring onions, chilli and coriander stalks in the processor until fine, then stir into the casserole pan • Roughly chop and add the tomatoes • Pour in the coconut milk, add the drained chickpeas, then tip in the pineapple chunks and their juices • Add the griddled cauliflower, cover, turn the heat up to high and bring to the boil

Put the uncooked poppadoms into the microwave (800W) for a minute or two to puff up • Tear off the top leafy half of the mint and bash to a paste in a pestle and mortar • Stir in the yoghurt, add a good squeeze of lemon juice and season with salt and pepper • Squeeze the juice of the remaining lemon into the curry and season to taste • Tear over the coriander leaves and serve with the rice and poppadoms

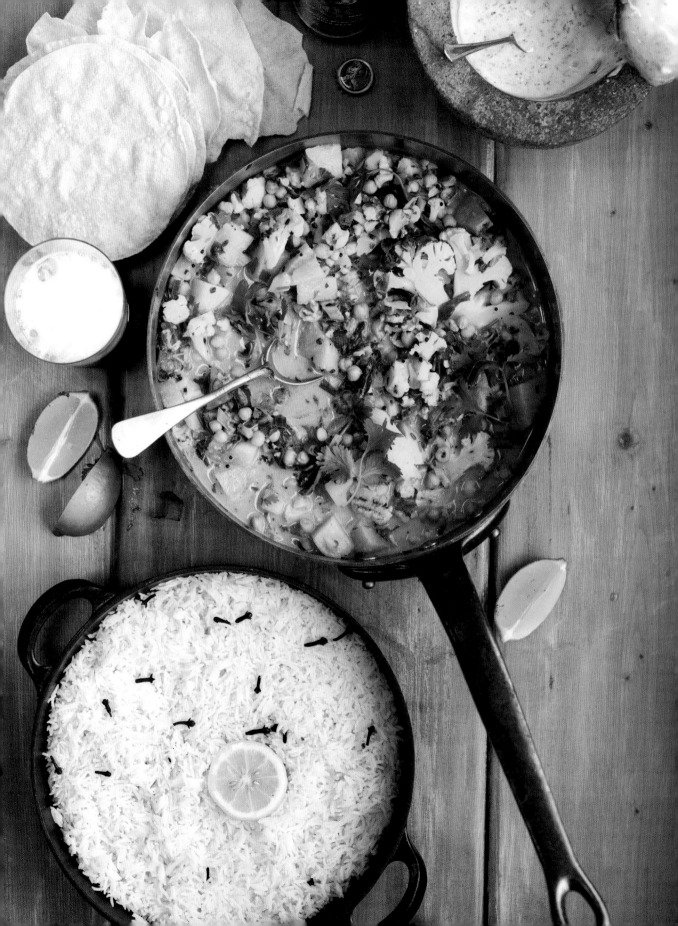

MODERN GREEK SALAD
SPINACH, CHICKPEA & FETA PARCELS

SERVES 4 | 516 CALORIES

Ingredients out • *Oven at 220°C/425°F/gas 7* • *Food processor (bowl blade, thick slicer & fine slicer)* • *Ovenproof medium frying pan, medium heat* • *Medium frying pan, medium heat*

Parcels
1 x 400g tin of chickpeas
100g feta cheese
100g baby spinach
1 lemon
½ tsp sweet smoked paprika
4 large sheets of filo pastry
  (from a 270g pack)
olive oil

Salad
1 cucumber
1 small red onion
½ a mixed bunch of fresh
  coriander and mint
20g blanched almonds
1 handful of black olives (stone in)
650g mixed ripe tomatoes
1 romaine lettuce
2 tbsp extra virgin olive oil

To serve
fat-free natural yoghurt
runny honey

START COOKING

Drain and add the chickpeas to the processor along with the feta, spinach, lemon zest and paprika, then blitz until combined • Fold a large sheet of filo pastry in half, dollop ¼ of the mixture into the centre, push your thumb into the middle to make a space for the filling to expand as it cooks, then bring the sides up and very loosely pinch into a parcel • Repeat to make 4 parcels • Add to the ovenproof pan with 1 tablespoon of olive oil and fry for a couple of minutes to crisp up the bottom, then bake in the oven until beautifully golden and crisp

Swap to the thick slicer in the processor • Scratch a fork down the length of the cucumber all the way round, then run it through the processor • Swap to the fine slicer and run through the peeled onion • Tip the veg into a bowl, season with salt, squeeze over the juice of the zested lemon and scrunch to mix • Finely chop and scatter over most of the top leafy half of the coriander and mint

Put the almonds and olives into the empty pan with 1 tablespoon of olive oil • Thickly slice the tomatoes and arrange nicely on a large platter • Slice the lettuce 1cm thick and add to the platter, then sprinkle over the cucumber and onion, drizzle with the extra virgin olive oil and spoon over the contents from the pan • Serve the parcels with a good dollop of yoghurt, a good drizzle of honey and the salad

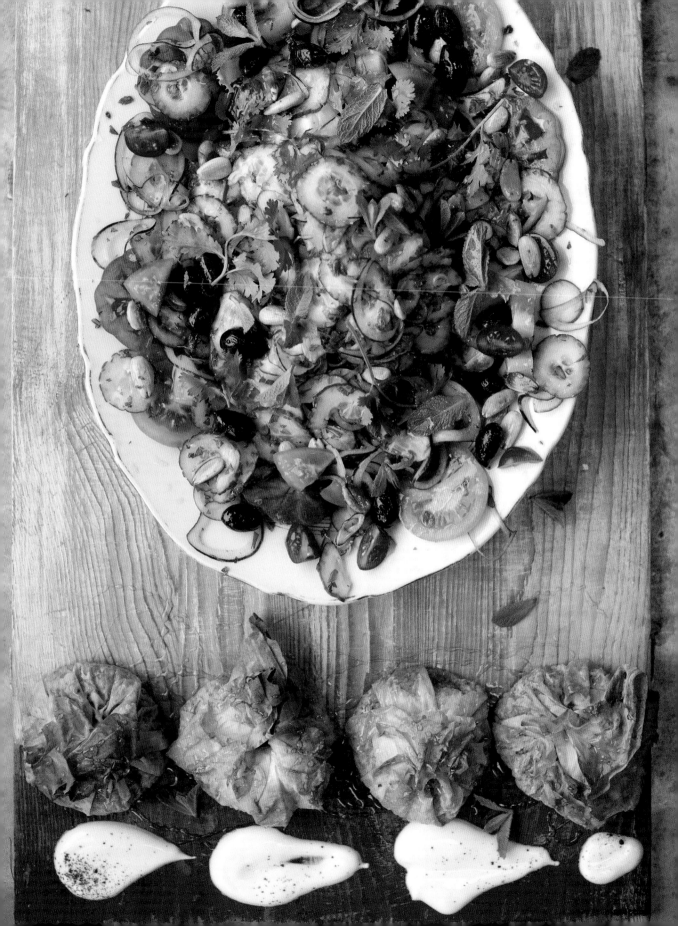

RICOTTA FRITTERS
TOMATO SAUCE & COURGETTE SALAD

SERVES 4 | 408 CALORIES

Ingredients out • Kettle boiled • Large frying pan, medium heat • Large casserole pan, low heat • Food processor (fine grater)

Sauce
25g dried porcini mushrooms
optional: 4 anchovy fillets
1 dried red chilli
2 cloves of garlic
700g passata
8 black olives (stone in)
½ a bunch of fresh basil

Fritters
1 large egg
400g ricotta cheese
1 whole nutmeg, for grating
1 lemon
40g Parmesan cheese
1 heaped tbsp plain flour
olive oil
balsamic vinegar

Salad
400g firm green or yellow
   baby courgettes
1 tbsp extra virgin olive oil
1 fresh red chilli
½ a bunch of fresh mint
1 lemon

START COOKING

Put the porcini into a mug and cover with boiling water • Crack the egg into a mixing bowl, add the ricotta, finely grate in ¼ of the nutmeg, the lemon zest and Parmesan, add the flour, then beat together • Put 1 tablespoon of olive oil into the frying pan, then use a tablespoon to spoon in 8 large dollops of the mixture, turning carefully when nice and golden

Put the anchovies (if using) and 1 tablespoon of olive oil into the casserole pan, crumble in the dried chilli, and squash in the unpeeled garlic through a garlic crusher • Finely chop and add the porcini with half their soaking water and the passata, season with salt and pepper and bring to the boil • Squash and add the olives, discarding the stones • Pick and reserve a few basil leaves, then chop the rest and add to the sauce

Grate the courgettes in the processor (you could use a box grater here) and tip into a bowl with a pinch of salt and pepper, the juice of the zested lemon and the extra virgin olive oil • Finely chop and add the chilli and the top leafy half of the mint, then toss together • Place the fritters on top of the sauce, then scatter over the reserved basil leaves, drizzle with balsamic and serve with lemon wedges

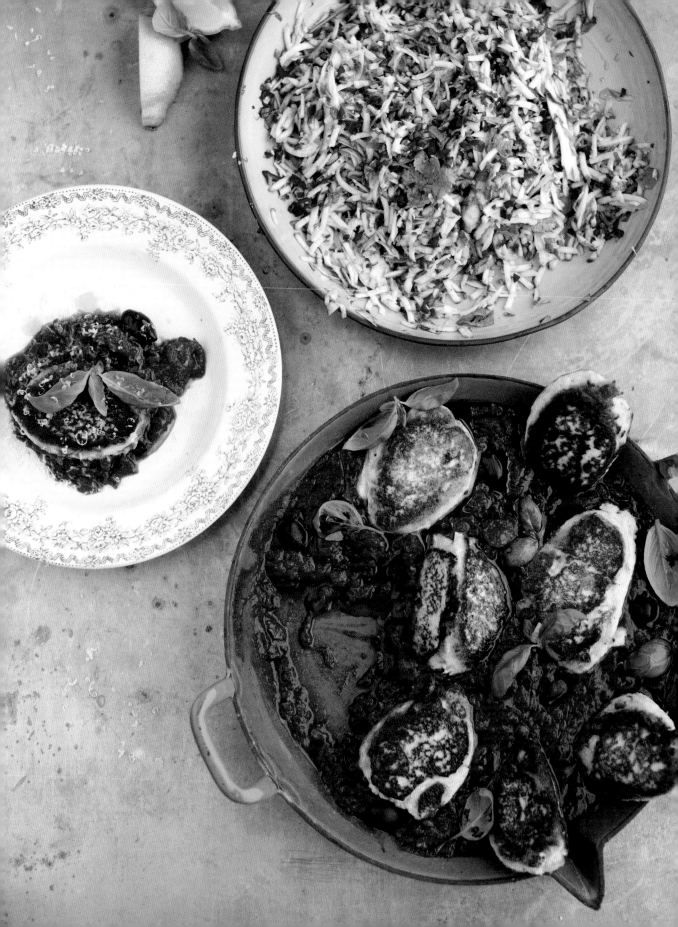

SWEET & SOUR VEGGIES
SCHEZUAN EGGY RICE & CRUNCH SALAD

SERVES 4 | 481 CALORIES

Ingredients out • Large frying pan, medium heat • Wok, medium heat • Food processor (coarse grater & fine slicer)

Rice
1 tsp Schezuan pepper
2 x 250g packs cooked brown rice
1 lemon
2 tbsp sweet chilli sauce
2 large eggs

Stir-fry
2 mixed-colour peppers
1 bunch of asparagus (300g)
1 fresh red chilli
1 thumb-sized piece of ginger
2 cloves of garlic
sesame oil
125g baby corn
1 bunch of fresh coriander
1 heaped tsp cornflour
1 x 227g tin pineapple chunks
   in juice
1 tbsp runny honey
2 tbsp sherry vinegar
200g beansprouts

Salad
2 carrots
200g sugar snap peas
1 bunch of fresh mint
1 lime
low-salt soy sauce

START COOKING

Crumble the Schezuan pepper and rice into the frying pan and squeeze in the lemon juice, tossing regularly • Tear the seeds and stalks out of the peppers and slice into 2cm chunks along with the trimmed asparagus • Finely chop the chilli, peeled ginger and garlic, then add to the wok with 2 tablespoons of oil • Add the peppers, asparagus and baby corn, tossing regularly

Roughly slice the coriander stalks and add to the wok (reserving the leaves) • Trim the carrots and coarsely grate in the processor • Swap to the fine slicer and run through the sugar snaps • Tip into a large bowl, rip off and toss through the top leafy half of the mint, then dress with the lime juice and 1 tablespoon of oil, and season to taste with soy sauce

Toss the cornflour with the veg in the wok, followed by the pineapple and juice, honey, vinegar and beansprouts • Toss well and season to taste with soy sauce • Push the rice to one side of the pan, then pour the chilli sauce into the space and let it bubble • Crack in the eggs and stir, gradually pulling in the rice • Serve everything sprinkled with coriander leaves

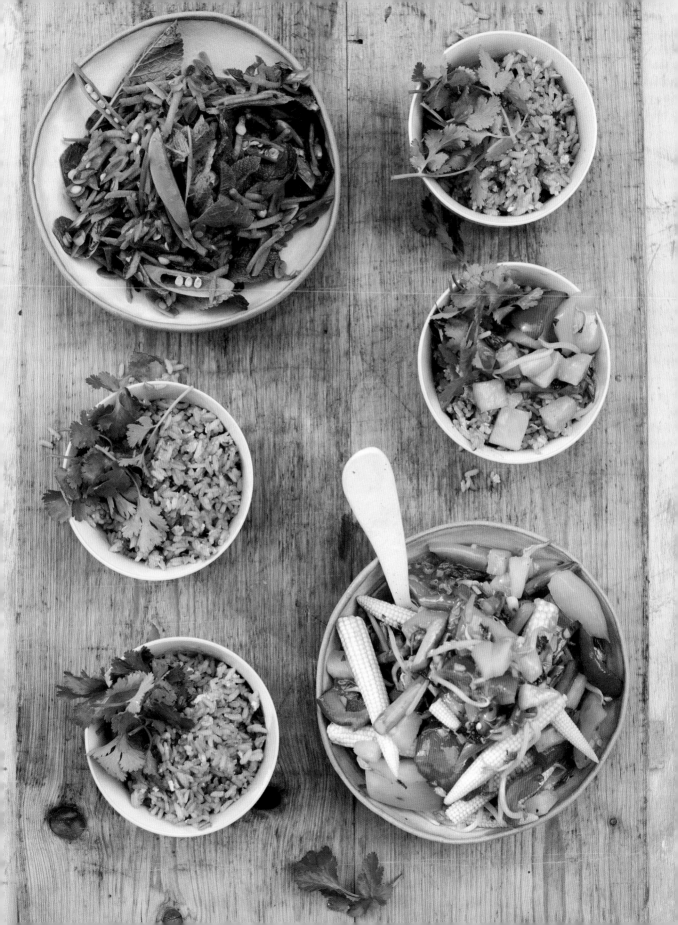

CAMEMBERT PARCELS
AUTUMN SALAD & CRANBERRY DIP

SERVES 4 | 651 CALORIES

Ingredients out • Food processor (bowl blade) • Large frying pan, medium heat • Small pan, medium heat • Liquidizer

Camembert parcels
200g Camembert cheese
100g shelled walnuts
1 bunch of fresh chives
1 lemon
4 large sheets of filo pastry
   (from a 270g pack)
1 tsp olive oil

Cranberry sauce
75g dried cranberries
1 pinch of ground cloves
½ tsp ground ginger
125ml port

Salad
1 pomegranate
2 tbsp balsamic vinegar
2 tbsp extra virgin olive oil
1 red chicory
1 green chicory
1 eating apple
100g watercress

START COOKING

Tear the Camembert into the processor with the walnuts and half the chives • Finely grate in the lemon zest and blitz until combined • On a clean surface, fold each sheet of pastry in half widthways • Add ¼ of the mixture across the bottom of one folded sheet in a sausage shape, push your thumb into the centre to make a space for the filling to expand as it cooks, and roll it up really loosely, like a long cigar • Repeat until you have 4 parcels • Rub each with olive oil and put into the frying pan, turning until golden and crispy

Put the cranberry sauce ingredients into the small pan with a splash of water and leave to bubble away • Halve the pomegranate and squeeze the juice from one half through your fingers on to a large platter • Add the balsamic, extra virgin olive oil, and a pinch of salt and pepper, then finely slice and scatter over the remaining chives • Finely slice the chicory bases and click the upper leaves apart • Coarsely grate or matchstick the apple, then add to the platter with the chicory and watercress

Blitz the cranberry mixture in the liquidizer until smooth (you may need to add a splash of water) • Pour on to a small platter or into a bowl and serve with the parcels for dipping • Toss the salad at the table, then hold the remaining pomegranate half cut side down over the salad and bash the back of it with a spoon so the seeds tumble on top

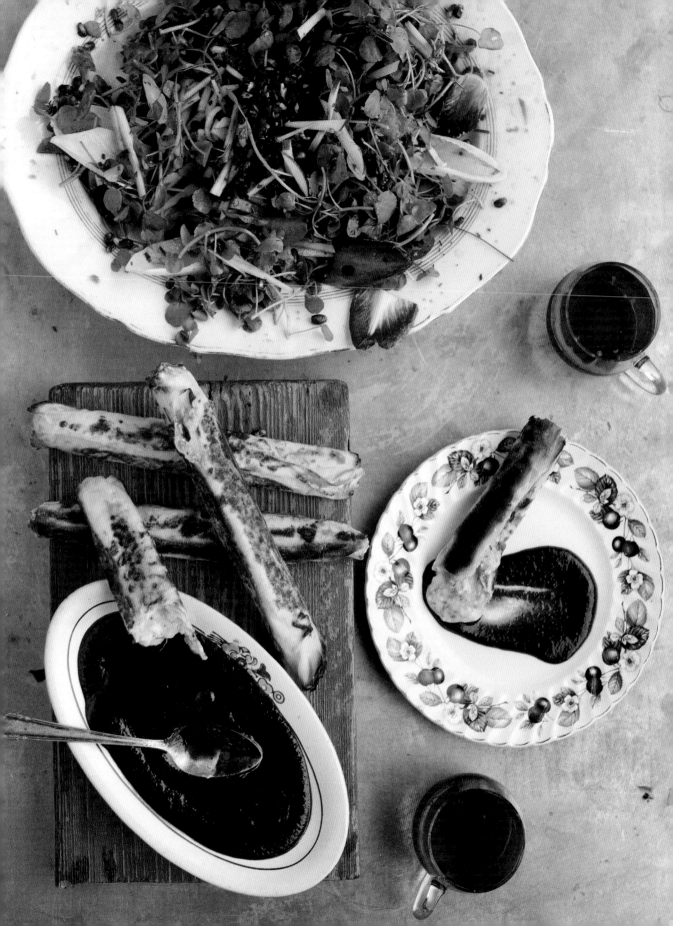

MEXICAN SALAD
CHARRED AVO & POPCORN BEANS

SERVES 4 | 725 CALORIES

Nachos

175g low-salt tortilla chips
30g Cheddar cheese
1 fresh red chilli
1 fresh green chilli

Salad

1 x 400g tin of kidney beans
1 x 400g tin of mixed beans
olive oil
1 pinch of ground cumin
2 ripe avocados
1 good pinch of ground coriander
200g mixed salad leaves

Dressing

2 spring onions
1 bunch of fresh coriander
1 tbsp jarred sliced jalapeños
extra virgin olive oil
2 tbsp fat-free natural yoghurt
2 limes

Ingredients out • Oven grill on medium • Medium frying pan, medium heat • Large griddle pan, high heat • Liquidizer

START COOKING

Spread the tortilla chips out in a roasting tray and grate over the Cheddar • Finely slice the chillies, sprinkle all over and pop under the grill on the middle shelf, removing when golden • Drain all the beans and tip into the frying pan with 1 tablespoon of olive oil and the cumin, tossing regularly until bursting open and crispy

Quarter, destone and peel the avocados, toss with 1 teaspoon of olive oil, salt, pepper and the ground coriander • Place them on the hot griddle until nicely charred all over, then remove • Trim and halve the spring onions, then blitz in the liquidizer with half the coriander, the jalapeños and a good splash of their vinegar, 1 tablespoon of extra virgin olive oil, the yoghurt and the juice of 1 lime, then pour into a bowl

Put the salad leaves into a nice serving bowl with the top leafy half of the remaining coriander, then arrange the charred avocado in and around the salad and scatter the popcorn beans over the top • Drizzle with 1 teaspoon of extra virgin olive oil, and serve with the cheesy chilli tortillas, lime wedges, and the dressing for dunking and drizzling

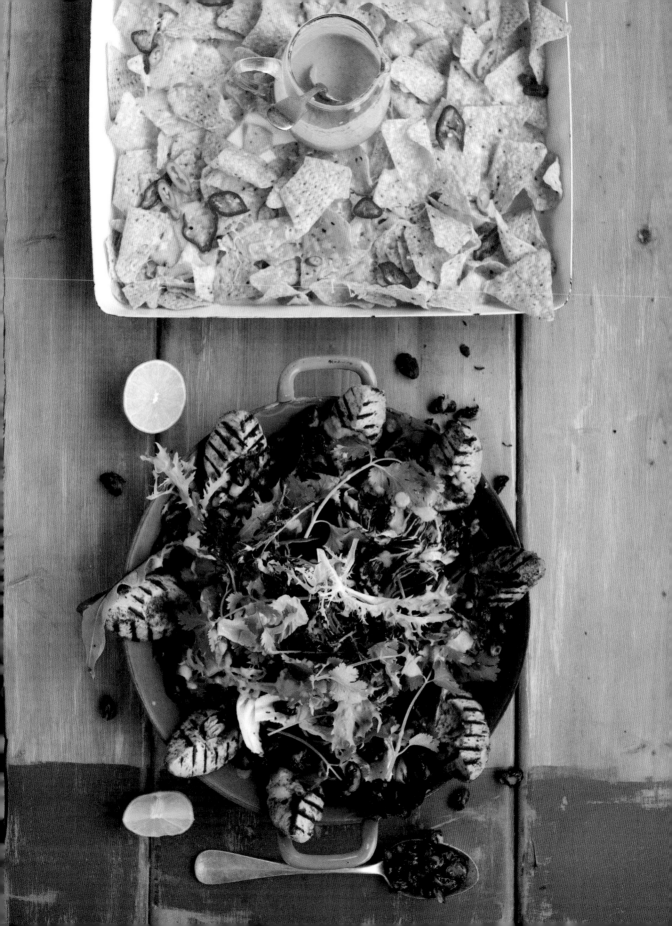

TASTY DAAL CURRY
WARM TOMATO SALAD & NAAN

SERVES 4 | 696 CALORIES

Ingredients out • *Kettle boiled* • *Oven at 130°C/250°F/gas ½* • *Food processor (bowl blade)* • *Lidded casserole pan, high heat* • *Frying pan, low heat*

Daal

1 onion
1 clove of garlic
1 thumb-sized piece of ginger
1–2 fresh red chillies
1 red pepper
1 big bunch of fresh coriander
rapeseed oil
1 handful of fresh curry leaves
1 tsp turmeric
1 tsp fenugreek seeds
2 tsp mustard seeds
300g dried red split lentils
1 x 400g tin of light coconut milk
200g baby spinach

Salad

500g ripe mixed-colour
   cherry tomatoes
1 lemon
1 tsp chilli powder
2 cloves of garlic

To serve

2 naan breads
fat-free natural yoghurt

START COOKING

Put the peeled onion halves, garlic and ginger, the chilli, deseeded pepper, coriander stalks and a pinch of salt and pepper into the processor, then blitz until fine • Put 1 tablespoon of oil into the casserole pan with the curry leaves, turmeric, fenugreek seeds and half the mustard seeds, and stir well • Add the blitzed veg and fry for a couple of minutes before adding the lentils, 700ml boiling water and the coconut milk • Put the lid on and boil, stirring regularly

Pop the naan breads in the oven • Halve the cherry tomatoes and finely chop half the lemon (rind and all) • Put 1 tablespoon of oil, the chilli powder, chopped lemon and remaining mustard seeds into the frying pan • Squash in the unpeeled garlic through a garlic crusher, squeeze over the remaining lemon juice, add the tomatoes and toss for 30 seconds, then season to taste

Fold the spinach through the daal, remove the naans from the oven, then take everything to the table with a bowl of yoghurt • Finish with a scattering of coriander leaves

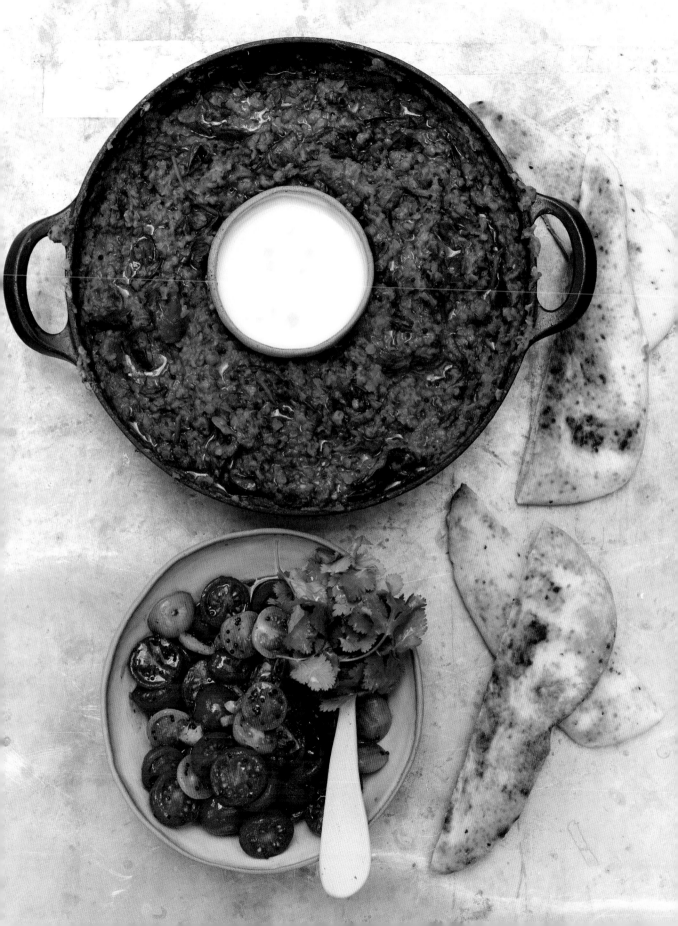

SPRING FRITTATA
TOMATO TOASTS, WATERCRESS & PEA SALAD

SERVES 4 | 468 CALORIES

Ingredients out • Oven grill on high • Food processor (fine grater & fine slicer)
• 26cm ovenproof frying pan, high heat • Griddle pan, high heat

Frittata

2 firm medium green
  or yellow courgettes
1 bunch of fresh mint
olive oil
8 large eggs
½ tsp truffle oil
1 pinch of cayenne pepper
4 sprigs of fresh thyme
40g pecorino cheese
1 fresh red chilli
20g feta cheese

Toasts

4 x 2cm slices of ciabatta
1 clove of garlic
4 ripe cherry tomatoes
1 tsp dried oregano

Salad

extra virgin olive oil
1 lemon
150g podded raw peas
100g watercress
1 celery heart

START COOKING

Grate the courgettes in the processor, put into a bowl, season well with salt, tear in a few mint leaves, then toss and squeeze to get rid of the excess salty liquid • Put 1 teaspoon of olive oil into the frying pan, sprinkle in the courgettes and fry for a few minutes, stirring often • Beat the eggs in a bowl with the truffle oil, cayenne, thyme leaves and half the finely grated pecorino, then pour the mixture over the courgettes • Stir and mix for a minute, then scatter over the rest of the grated pecorino and put on the top shelf under the grill until cooked through, fluffy and golden (roughly 5 minutes)

Put the ciabatta slices on the griddle pan, turning when golden • Pour 2 tablespoons of extra virgin olive oil on to a serving platter with the lemon juice and a pinch of salt and pepper • Roughly chop the rest of the leafy top half of the mint and scatter over the platter with the peas and watercress • Swap to the fine slicer in the processor, then remove the outer celery sticks (save for another day), slice just the bottom half of the heart and add to the salad with the finely sliced leafy tops

Remove the toasts to a nice serving board, rub each one with the cut side of the garlic and squash in a tomato, then sprinkle with oregano and 1 teaspoon of extra virgin olive oil • Finely slice the chilli, then slide the frittata on to the board, scatter with the chilli, crumble over the feta and serve with the salad, tossing gently at the last minute

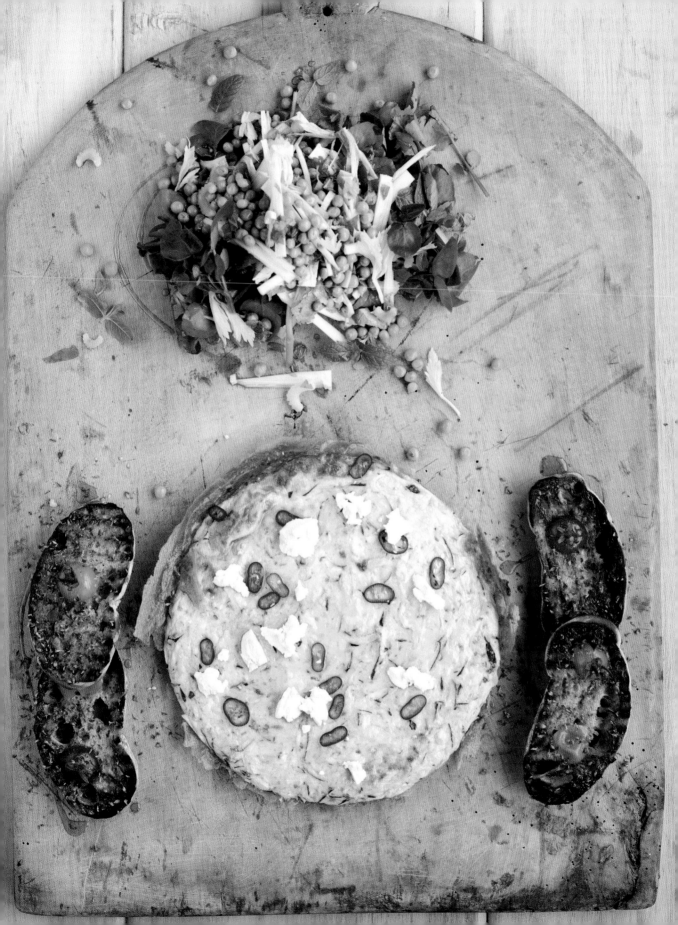

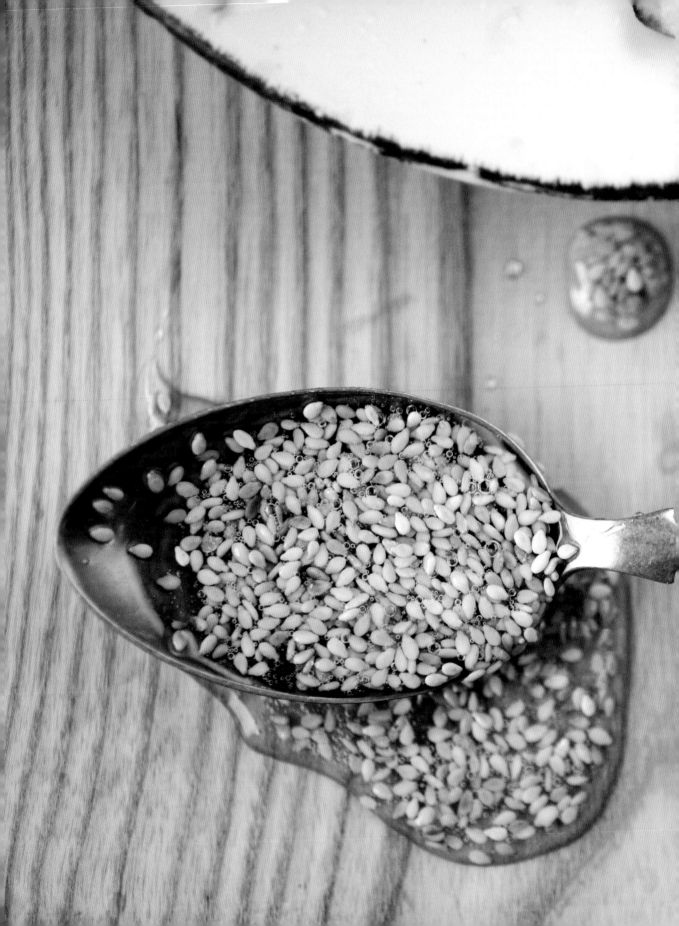

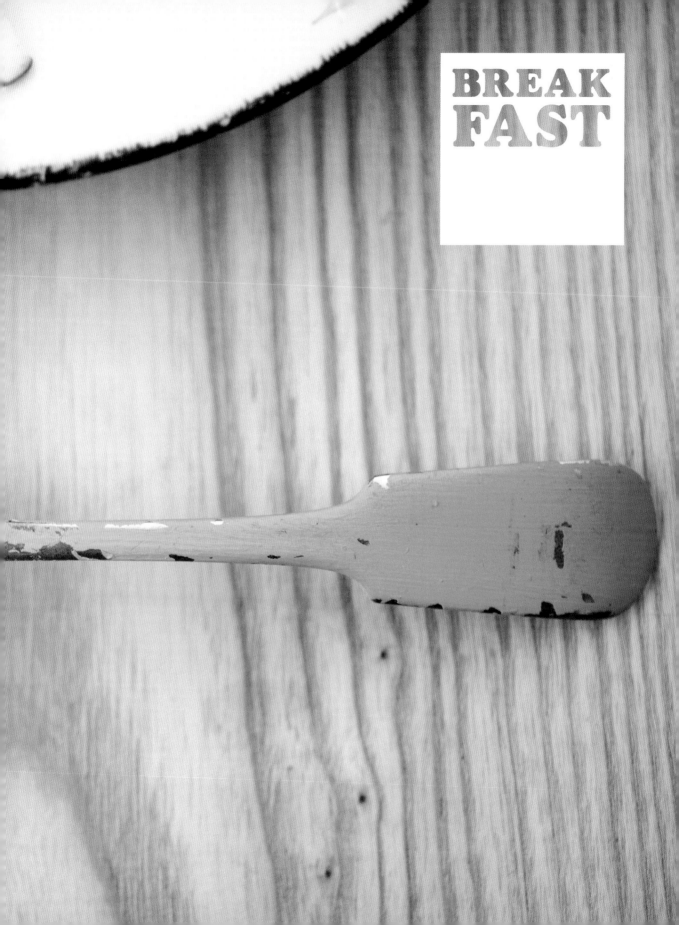

BREAK
FAST

SMOKY MAPLE PANCETTA
FLUFFY CORN & CHILLI PANCAKES

SERVES 4 | 477 CALORIES

Pancakes

1 cup of self-raising flour
1 large egg
1 cup of semi-skimmed milk
1 fresh green chilli
40g Cheddar cheese
1 handful of frozen sweetcorn
olive oil

Toppings

4 ripe tomatoes
1 ripe avocado
1 lime
½ a bunch of fresh coriander
8 rashers of smoked pancetta
maple syrup
4 tbsp fat-free natural yoghurt
Lingham's chilli sauce

This is an amazing weekend breakfast – it will put a smile on your face, get you going and make you feel really satisfied. A hit of chilli wakes you up better than any espresso, trust me.

START COOKING

Whisk the flour, egg and milk in a bowl with a pinch of salt until smooth • Finely slice the chilli, grate the cheese, then fold both into the batter with the sweetcorn • Roughly chop the tomatoes and the peeled, destoned avocado, then toss with the juice from ½ a lime, the top leafy half of the coriander, salt and pepper

Put the pancetta into a medium frying pan on a medium-low heat, turning when crisp and golden • Drizzle with maple syrup, glaze for 20 seconds, then remove from the heat • Drizzle 1 teaspoon of oil into a small frying pan on a medium heat, add a ladleful of batter and spread it out to the edges • Flip when golden and remove to a plate once done

Place ¼ of the topping and pancetta on top of the pancake and serve with a dollop of yoghurt, a wedge of lime, and chilli sauce if you like that extra hit • Repeat with the remaining ingredients and serve as and when they're ready

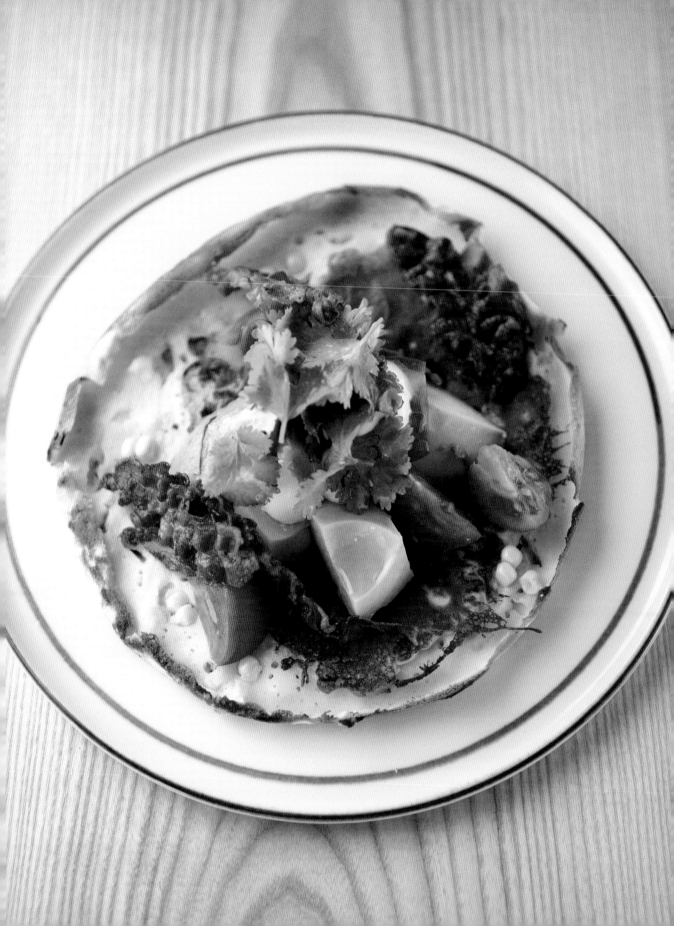

AVOCADO ON TOAST
FOUR WAYS

SERVES 1 | 269 CALORIES

AVO & EGG

Fill and boil the kettle • Toast **1 slice of nice bread** • Get a small pan on a high heat, fill it with boiling water and add a **pinch of salt** • Swirl the water with a fork, then crack in **1 large super-fresh egg** and poach to your liking • Destone, peel and slice **½ a ripe avocado** • Halve **1 ripe cherry tomato** and rub into the toast, then drizzle with **1 teaspoon of extra virgin olive oil** • Cover with the avocado and scatter with **a few slices of fresh red chilli** • Pop your egg on top, bust it open and season to taste

SERVES 1 | 268 CALORIES

AVO & CRISPY PANCETTA

Grill **3 rashers of smoked pancetta** on a hot griddle pan, with **1 slice of nice bread** on the side to soak up the tasty fat • Destone and peel **½ a ripe avocado** • Turn the toast and use a fork to squash the avocado into it, spreading it right to the edges • Add **a little pinch of salt and pepper**, **a squeeze of lime** or **lemon juice, a few slices of fresh red chilli** and **4 fresh basil leaves**, then serve with the crispy pancetta on top

SERVES 1 | 256 CALORIES

AVO & SMOKED HAM

Toast **1 slice of nice bread** • Drizzle it with **1 teaspoon of olive oil**, then lay **1 slice of ripe beef tomato** and **1 slice of cooked ham** on top • Destone and peel **½ a ripe avocado** and place on top, then add **a little pinch of salt and pepper** and squeeze **lime** or **lemon juice** into the well with a few drips of oil • Use a speed-peeler to peel over **10g Emmental cheese**, then scatter with **4 fresh basil leaves**

SERVES 1 | 303 CALORIES

AVO & SMOKED SALMON

Toast **1 slice of nice bread** • Drizzle it with **1 teaspoon of extra virgin olive oil** and cover with **35g smoked salmon** • Use a teaspoon to add small bombs of **cream cheese (25g in total)** on top • Destone **½ a ripe avocado**, then use a teaspoon to curl small nuggets of the flesh over the toast • Finely grate over **a little lemon zest**, then add a squeeze of juice and **a pinch of pepper**

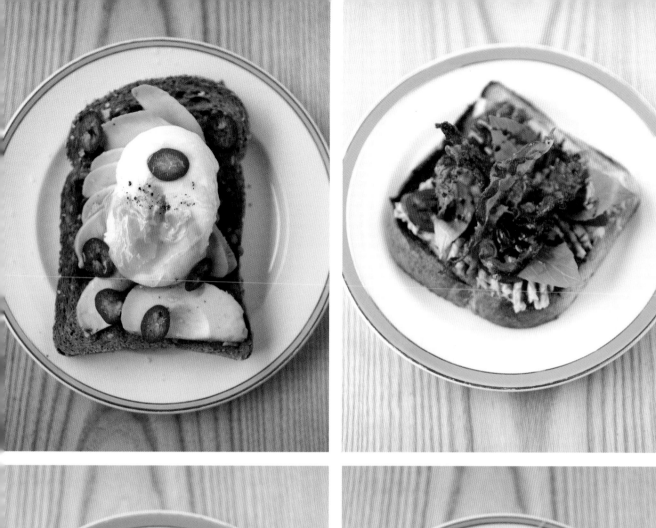
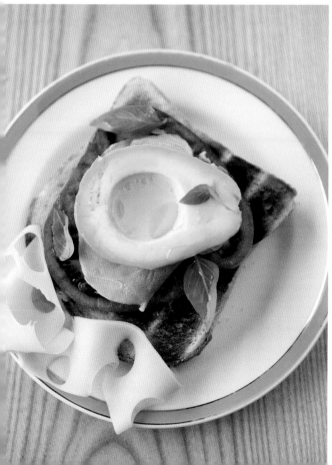
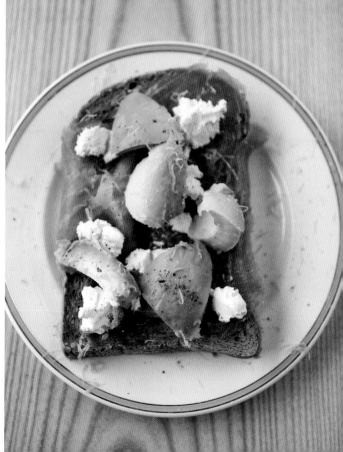

BRING BACK THE TOASTIE
(PART 1: HOT SANDWICH HEAVEN)

SERVES 1 | 384 CALORIES

2 fresh chives
2 slices of bread
2 slices of smoked salmon
1 large egg
10g Cheddar cheese

SMOKED SALMON & EGG

Chop the chives • Place 1 piece of bread in a toastie maker and drape the smoked salmon in a circle on top, leaving a gap in the middle where you can crack in the egg • Scatter over the chopped chives, finely grate over the Cheddar and season with salt and pepper • Carefully top with the second piece of bread and toast away

SERVES 1 | 310 CALORIES

2 slices of bread
1 ripe tomato
30g feta cheese
¼ of an avocado
2 pinches of dried oregano

GREEK-STYLE

Place 1 piece of bread in a toastie maker, then slice and add the tomato • Crumble over the feta • Peel and roughly chop the avocado, pile on top and scatter with a pinch of oregano • Top with the second piece of bread, scatter with the remaining oregano and toast away

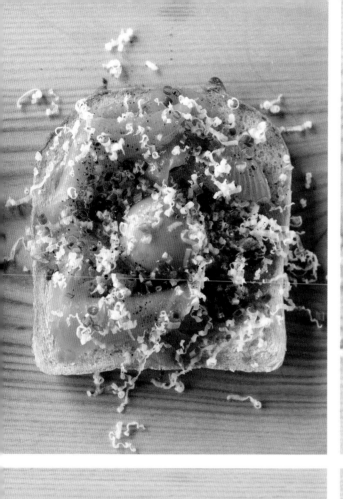
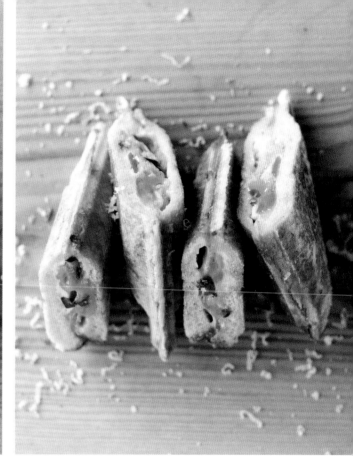
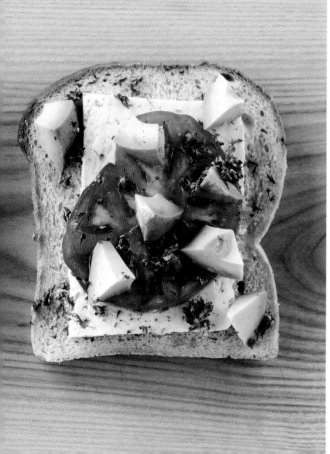
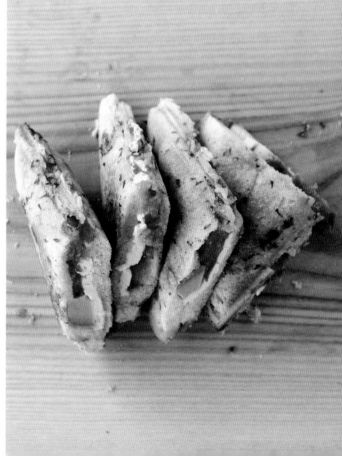

VIVA LA TOASTIE
(PART 2: SOME MORE HOT OPTIONS)

2 slices of bread
25g Cheddar cheese
3 button mushrooms
1 small handful of rocket
¼ of a lemon
20g cured chorizo sausage

CLASSIC CHEESE & MUSHROOM

Place 1 piece of bread in a toastie maker, then grate over the cheese • Slice and lay over the mushrooms • Chop the rocket, toss in the lemon juice and pile on top, then top with the second piece of bread • Finely slice the chorizo, lay on the top of the sandwich, clamp down well so they stick together, and toast away

25g ricotta cheese
1 heaped tsp runny honey
20g dark chocolate
   (70% cocoa solids)
1 small banana
2 slices of bread

SWEET NAUGHTY BEGINNING

Beat the ricotta with the honey, smash the chocolate, and peel and roughly chop the banana • Place 1 piece of bread in a toastie maker, then spread the ricotta on top • Lay over the banana and scatter over the chocolate • Top with the second piece of bread and toast away

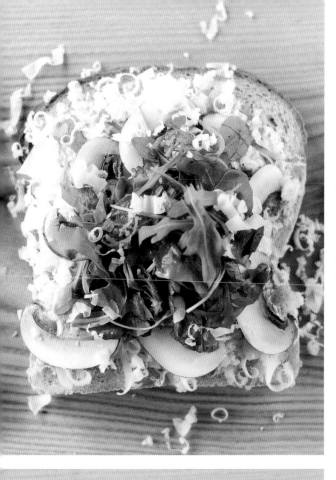 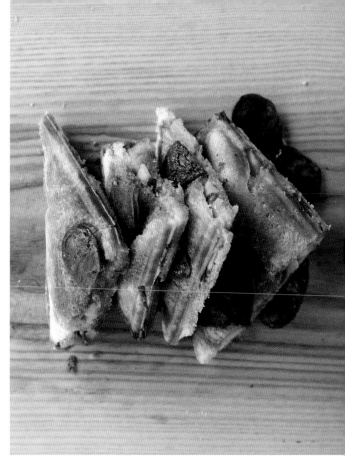

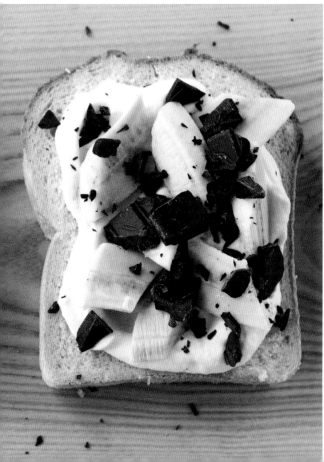 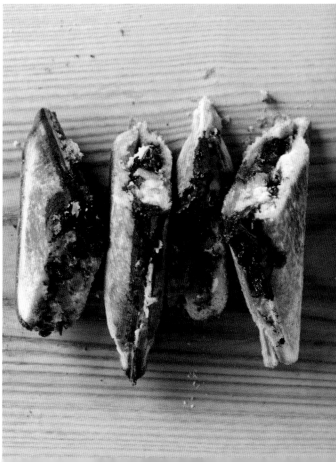

FANTASTIC GRANOLA
GET UP, GET FED, GET GONE

MAKES 3 x 1 LITRE JARS | 332 CALORIES

Granola mix

100g Brazil nuts

100g shelled walnuts

100g shelled pistachios

100g pumpkin seeds

100g sunflower seeds

100g sesame seeds

500g porridge oats

40g desiccated coconut

1 tsp ground cinnamon

75g sour cherries

250g dried apricots

To serve

maple syrup

milk or fat-free natural yoghurt

My suggestion is to buy a big batch of ingredients like the list I've given you here, mix it all up and just grab a handful per person whenever you need it – it will last for months. I love it served with fresh blueberries or pomegranate seeds.

START COOKING

Roughly bash up the nuts and seeds in a pestle and mortar or pulse them in a food processor with a bowl blade – I like some fine and some chunky • Mix them with the smashed nuts and seeds, oats, coconut and cinnamon

Now you've got a choice: you can either mix it with the chopped cherries and apricots and decant it straight into airtight jars to toast as and when you want it, or you can spread it across a couple of large roasting trays and toast it in a preheated oven at 180°C/350°F/gas 4 until nicely golden, stirring regularly • Let it cool, then mix in the chopped cherries and apricots and tip into jars to await eating

If you want to toast it as and when you want it, I just put a dry frying pan on a medium heat and add a handful of granola (roughly 50g) per person • Toast for 3 or so minutes, tossing often to bring out the roasted flavour and crispy texture, until lightly golden and smelling delicious • Stir in a good teaspoon of maple syrup per person and let it get sticky, then serve hot with cold milk or yoghurt and fresh seasonal fruit, if you like

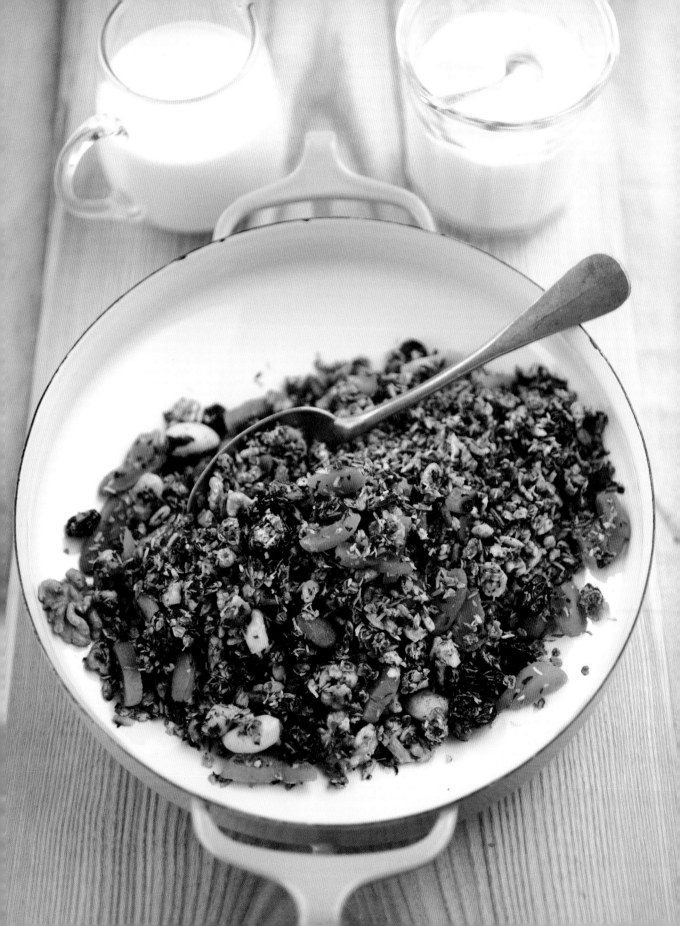

SUPERB BOX GRATER
FRUIT SALAD

SERVES 4 | 91 CALORIES

Sesame honey
1 handful of sesame seeds
½ a small jar of runny honey

Ripe fruit
1 pear
1 nectarine
1 handful of strawberries
1 banana
1 apple

Dressing
1 orange or lime
a couple of sprigs of fresh mint

To serve
fat-free natural yoghurt

This delicious breakfast is simplicity to the hilt, but don't be misled by that. It's beautiful, tasty, and the action of bruising and grating brings out all the natural sugars in the fruit, creating a liquor that gives it shine and juice. Couple that with the warm sesame honey and it's unbelievable. Definitely give it a go.

START COOKING

Toast the sesame seeds in a dry pan, tossing frequently until golden • Mix with the honey, then warm through in the microwave (800W) for 20 seconds before using • Keep the rest for another day – it's delicious and lasts a long time

Set up a box grater on a plate, then in long strokes coarsely and carefully grate all the fruit, piece by piece – you can use any slightly firm stone fruit like plums, peaches and nectarines, perfect orchard fruit, strawberries and bananas • Carefully lift off the grater, leaving a lovely pile of grated fruit • Squeeze over the orange or lime juice and drizzle with 2 tablespoons of sesame honey • Roughly chop the mint leaves and sprinkle over, then serve with natural yoghurt

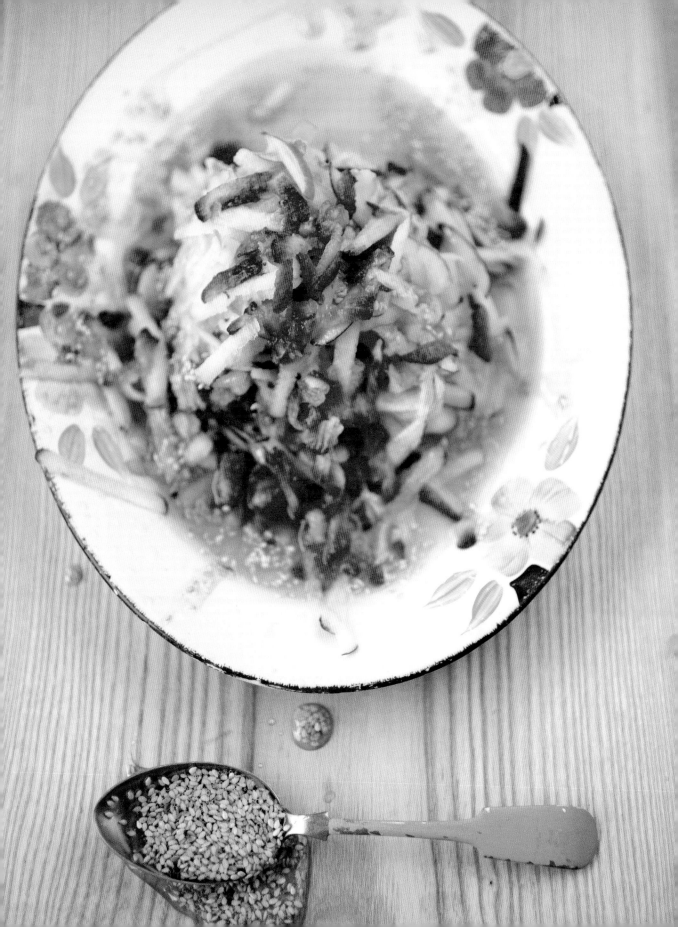

FRUIT 'N' NUT COMBOS
SWEETENED COTTAGE CHEESE

SERVES 6 | 189 CALORIES

This is about embracing beautiful combinations of simple ingredients for an instant breakfast. A 50g serving of sweetened cheese per person is more than enough, and if you're not feeding six, the sweetened cheese will keep well in the fridge for a couple of days.

START COOKING

In a bowl, mix **1 tablespoon of runny honey** and **1 heaped teaspoon of vanilla paste** into **300g cottage cheese or ricotta** (Greek yoghurt is also delicious) • Loosen with a **splash of milk** if needed and whip up, then divide between your plates or bowls • Top with wonderful **fresh fruit** like chopped mango, strawberries and watermelon, **a little squeeze of lime juice** and a scattering of **chopped** or **bashed shelled nuts** like Brazils, almonds or pistachios

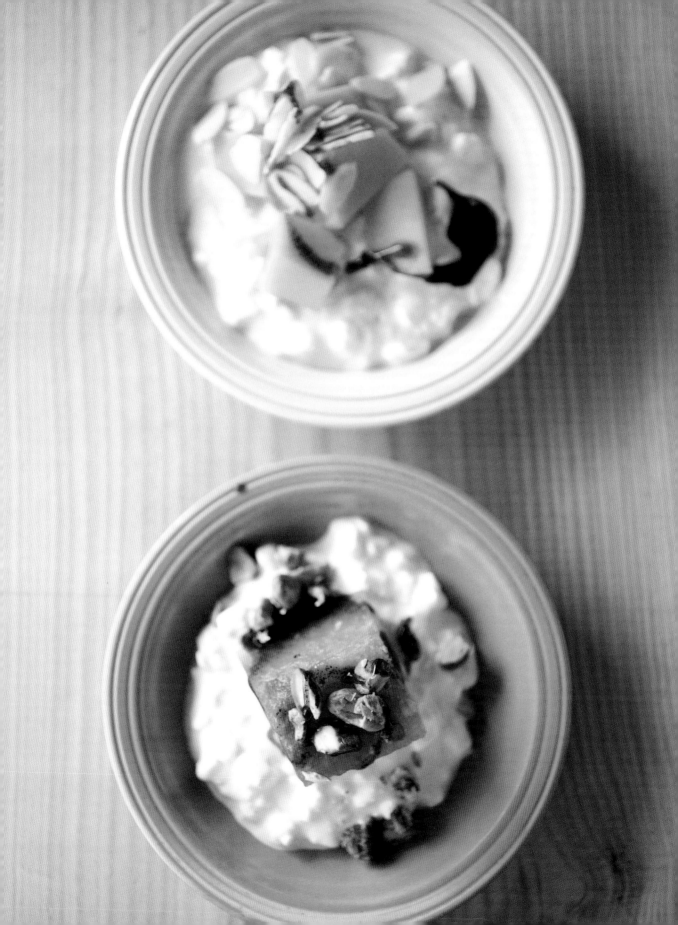

SUPER SMOOTHIES
FOUR WAYS TO KICK START YOUR DAY

You can make all these smoothies with fresh fruit, but what I like to do is bag up fruit combos and freeze them ahead of when I need them, which eliminates the need to add ice. This will also give you a thicker, even more delicious, cold smoothie that's guaranteed to invigorate and wake you up in the morning.

You can get brilliant frozen fruit from the supermarkets, but with things like bananas, or when there's a glut of seasonal fruit, get into the habit of bagging them up and freezing them yourself. Two minutes of thought one day will save you time every morning for a month, mean you've got treats in the freezer and can even save you money – if you've got fruit that's on the turn and you're not going to eat it, you can freeze it before it goes too far.

GREEN

146 CALORIES

In a liquidizer, blitz **1 large peeled banana** (ideally pre-chopped and frozen) with **200g baby spinach, 250ml fresh apple juice** and the **juice from 1 lime**, until smooth

PURPLE

100 CALORIES

Roughly chop **2 pears (stalks removed)**, put into a liquidizer with **150g frozen blueberries** and **100ml fresh apple juice**, then blitz until smooth

ORANGE

113 CALORIES

Finely grate **a 2cm piece of peeled ginger** into a liquidizer • Peel, trim, roughly chop and add **1 carrot**, and squeeze in the **juice of 1 lime** • Add **1 small frozen chopped mango** and **200ml fresh orange juice**, then blitz until smooth

WHITE

340 CALORIES

In a liquidizer, blitz **1 large peeled banana** (ideally pre-chopped and frozen) with **3 tablespoons of ground almonds, 250ml semi-skimmed milk** and **1 tablespoon of runny honey**, until smooth

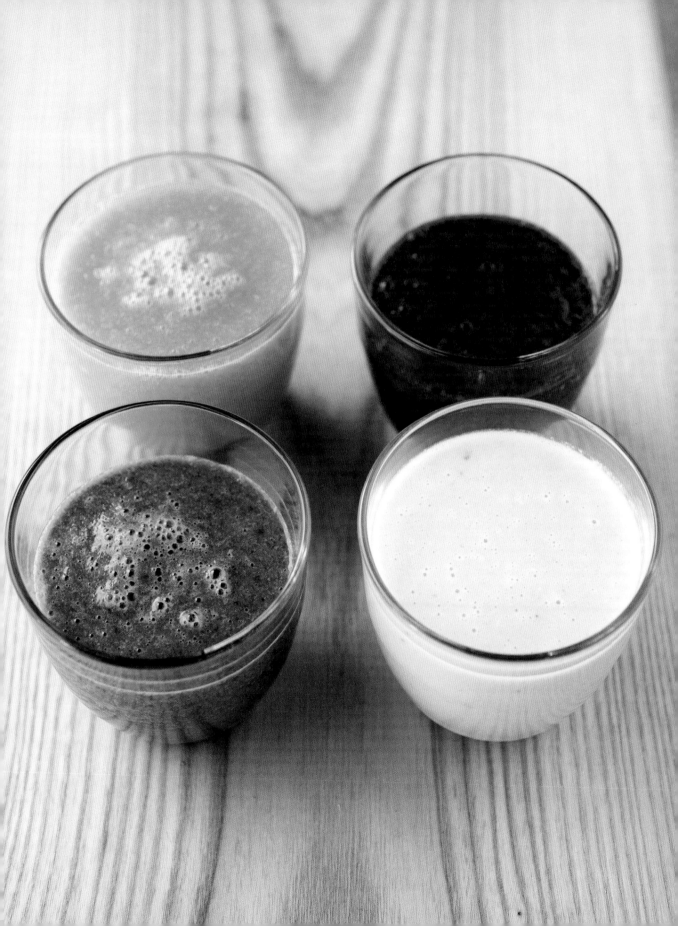

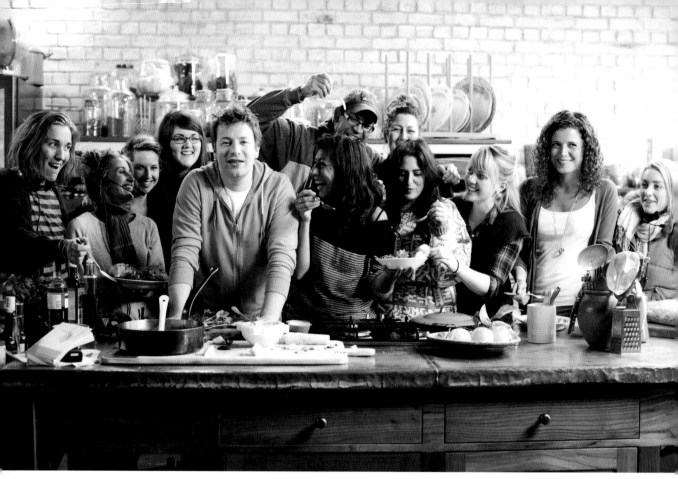

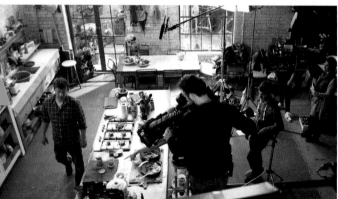

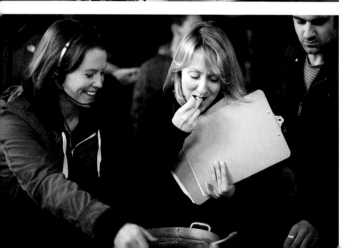

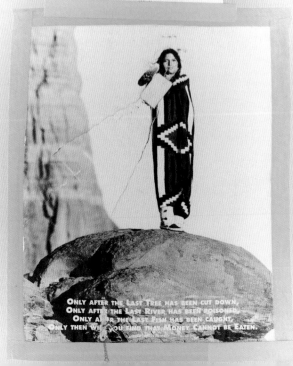

BEAUTIFUL THINGS HAPPEN WHEN YOU SMILE

ONLY AFTER THE LAST TREE HAS BEEN CUT DOWN,
ONLY AFTER THE LAST RIVER HAS BEEN POISONED,
ONLY AFTER THE LAST FISH HAS BEEN CAUGHT,
ONLY THEN WILL YOU FIND THAT MONEY CANNOT BE EATEN.

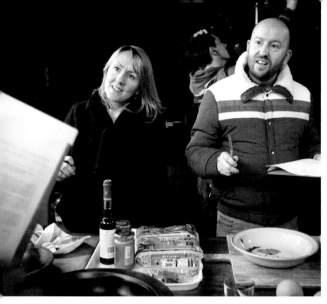
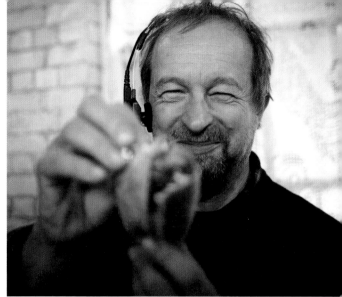
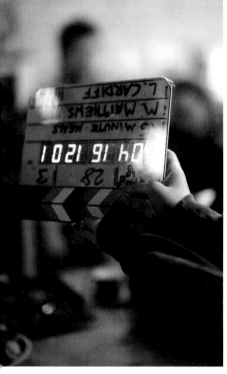
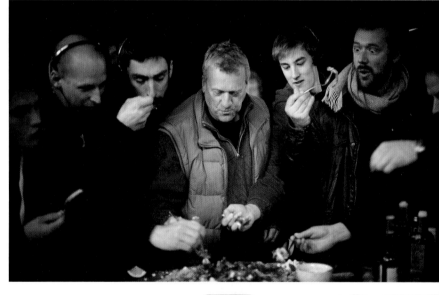
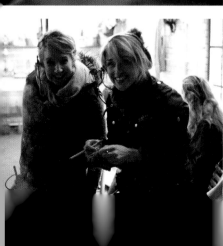
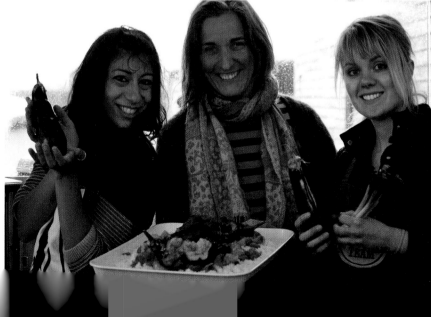

A NOTE ON NUTRITION
FROM LAURA PARR – JAMIE'S HEAD NUTRITIONIST

JAMIE AND I HAVE WORKED TOGETHER ON THIS BOOK TO CREATE RECIPES THAT DELIVER TASTY, GOOD-FOR-YOU FOOD, BUT DON'T COMPROMISE ON FLAVOUR. THIS ISN'T A DIET BOOK, BUT THE RECIPES HAVE BEEN WRITTEN MINDFULLY TO ACHIEVE A BALANCE BETWEEN CARBOHYDRATES, FRUIT AND/OR VEG, DAIRY AND PROTEIN, WITH THE ODD TREAT RECIPE THROWN IN (THIS IS REAL LIFE AFTER ALL!).

In the UK, all foods belong to one of the five food groups. These are:

- fruit and vegetables
- starchy carbohydrates such as bread, rice, potatoes and pasta
- meat, fish, eggs, beans and other non-dairy sources of protein
- milk and dairy foods
- food/drinks high in fat and/or sugar.

It's crucial to strike the right balance between the food and drink we consume from these groups every day. In a typical meal, we should aim for one-third fruit and vegetables and one-third carbohydrates, with the final one-third split between protein, dairy and a small amount of foods high in fat and/or sugar. This is what we've set out to achieve with the majority of these meals – obviously you don't have to have that balance in every single meal you eat, but it is a good guide to aim for on a day-to-day basis.

Eating treats is a part of life, but it's also important to recognize when we're pushing things too far, so we can redress the balance at other meals and get back on track. When we eat and drink, we're putting energy (calories) into our bodies, and understanding the amount of calories we consume is one way of monitoring our food intake in order to try and maintain a healthy weight. We've given you the calorie content per serving of every recipe in this book to encourage you to start thinking about how each of these meals fits into your daily calorie intake. As a guide, the average man needs around 2,500 calories a day to maintain a healthy body weight, and the average woman needs 2,000 calories a day.

By eating a wide range of different foods, you'll stand a greater chance of getting all the nutrients you need. So when you're cooking from this book, just mix up the recipes you choose, picking from all the different chapters. Of course you'll have your favourites, but try to eat a diverse mix – maybe fish a couple of nights a week (go for oily fish like sardines or mackerel once a week), a meat-free recipe on one or two nights, then a variety of beef, pork, lamb or chicken on the rest.

If you feel you need to make a few changes, here are some general tips to help you on your way to a healthier lifestyle. Use these as a rough guide and you'll be heading in the right direction to making better choices:

- Base your meals on starchy foods and include one-third potatoes, pasta, rice, quinoa, couscous or bread, choosing wholegrain varieties when you can.
- Eat lots of fruit and vegetables as they provide important vitamins and minerals.
- Eat more fish, and aim to have oily fish once a week.
- Cut down on saturated fat and sugar.
- Try to eat less salt – taste your food before seasoning it, as you can always add more salt but you can't take it away. And don't forget a lot of food already has salt in it, so really think about whether you need to add more or not.
- Drink plenty of water.
- Don't skip breakfast.
- Be as active as possible and aim to maintain a healthy weight.

Above all, enjoy the recipes in this book!

Don't forget, it's vital to balance the amount you eat with your level of activity, as different people have different nutritional requirements, depending on factors such as their age, gender and lifestyle.

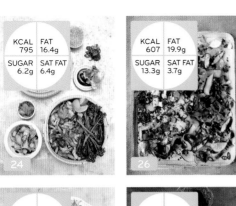

KCAL 795 | FAT 16.4g
SUGAR 6.2g | SAT FAT 6.4g

24

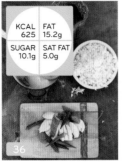

KCAL 607 | FAT 19.9g
SUGAR 13.3g | SAT FAT 3.7g

26

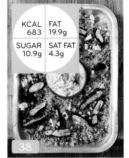

KCAL 651 | FAT 18.4g
SUGAR 17.8g | SAT FAT 4.0g

28

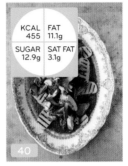

KCAL 557 | FAT 22.5g
SUGAR 4.4g | SAT FAT 3.3g

30

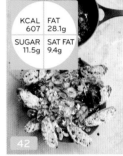

KCAL 610 | FAT 19.3g
SUGAR 10.4g | SAT FAT 4.5g

32

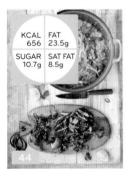

KCAL 694 | FAT 33.3g
SUGAR 17.1g | SAT FAT 7.1g

34

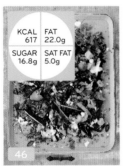

KCAL 625 | FAT 15.2g
SUGAR 10.1g | SAT FAT 5.0g

36

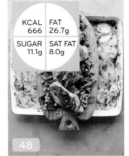

KCAL 683 | FAT 19.9g
SUGAR 10.9g | SAT FAT 4.3g

38

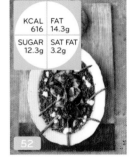

KCAL 455 | FAT 11.1g
SUGAR 12.9g | SAT FAT 3.1g

40

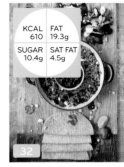

KCAL 607 | FAT 28.1g
SUGAR 11.5g | SAT FAT 9.4g

42

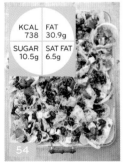

KCAL 656 | FAT 23.5g
SUGAR 10.7g | SAT FAT 8.5g

44

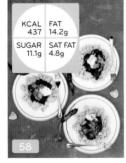

KCAL 617 | FAT 22.0g
SUGAR 16.8g | SAT FAT 5.0g

46

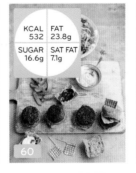

KCAL 666 | FAT 26.7g
SUGAR 11.1g | SAT FAT 8.0g

48

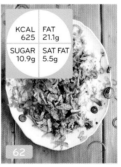

KCAL 476 | FAT 15.2g
SUGAR 10.3g | SAT FAT 4.7g

50

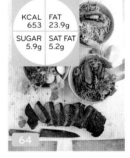

KCAL 616 | FAT 14.3g
SUGAR 12.3g | SAT FAT 3.2g

52

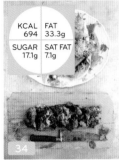

KCAL 738 | FAT 30.9g
SUGAR 10.5g | SAT FAT 6.5g

54

KCAL 437 | FAT 14.2g
SUGAR 11.1g | SAT FAT 4.8g

58

KCAL 532 | FAT 23.8g
SUGAR 16.6g | SAT FAT 7.1g

60

KCAL 625 | FAT 21.1g
SUGAR 10.9g | SAT FAT 5.5g

62

KCAL 653 | FAT 23.9g
SUGAR 5.9g | SAT FAT 5.2g

64

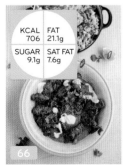

KCAL 706 | FAT 21.1g
SUGAR 9.1g | SAT FAT 7.6g

66

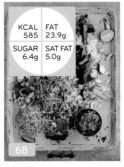

KCAL 585 | FAT 23.9g
SUGAR 6.4g | SAT FAT 5.0g

68

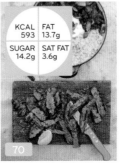

KCAL 593 | FAT 13.7g
SUGAR 14.2g | SAT FAT 3.6g

70

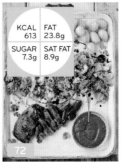

KCAL 613 | FAT 23.8g
SUGAR 7.3g | SAT FAT 8.9g

72

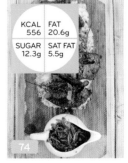

KCAL 556 | FAT 20.6g
SUGAR 12.3g | SAT FAT 5.5g

74

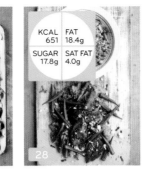
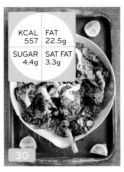
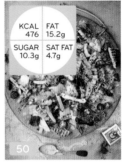

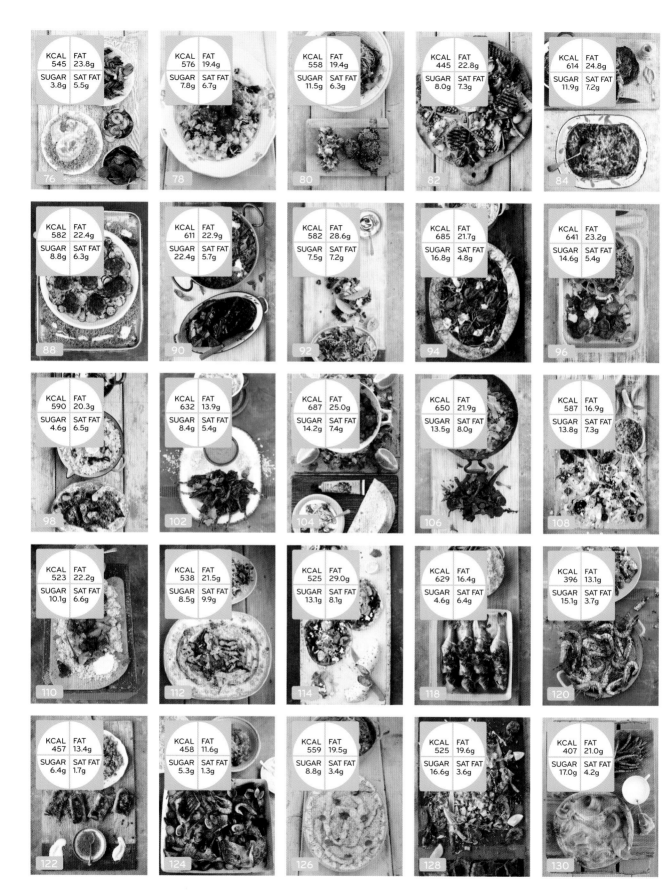

76	KCAL 545	FAT 23.8g	SUGAR 3.8g	SAT FAT 5.5g
78	KCAL 576	FAT 19.4g	SUGAR 7.8g	SAT FAT 6.7g
80	KCAL 558	FAT 19.4g	SUGAR 11.5g	SAT FAT 6.3g
82	KCAL 445	FAT 22.8g	SUGAR 8.0g	SAT FAT 7.3g
84	KCAL 614	FAT 24.8g	SUGAR 11.9g	SAT FAT 7.2g
88	KCAL 582	FAT 22.4g	SUGAR 8.8g	SAT FAT 6.3g
90	KCAL 611	FAT 22.9g	SUGAR 22.4g	SAT FAT 5.7g
92	KCAL 582	FAT 28.6g	SUGAR 7.5g	SAT FAT 7.2g
94	KCAL 685	FAT 21.7g	SUGAR 16.8g	SAT FAT 4.8g
96	KCAL 641	FAT 23.2g	SUGAR 14.6g	SAT FAT 5.4g
98	KCAL 590	FAT 20.3g	SUGAR 4.6g	SAT FAT 6.5g
102	KCAL 632	FAT 13.9g	SUGAR 8.4g	SAT FAT 5.4g
104	KCAL 687	FAT 25.0g	SUGAR 14.2g	SAT FAT 7.4g
106	KCAL 650	FAT 21.9g	SUGAR 13.5g	SAT FAT 8.0g
108	KCAL 587	FAT 16.9g	SUGAR 13.8g	SAT FAT 7.3g
110	KCAL 523	FAT 22.2g	SUGAR 10.1g	SAT FAT 6.6g
112	KCAL 538	FAT 21.5g	SUGAR 8.5g	SAT FAT 9.9g
114	KCAL 525	FAT 29.0g	SUGAR 13.1g	SAT FAT 8.1g
118	KCAL 629	FAT 16.4g	SUGAR 4.6g	SAT FAT 6.4g
120	KCAL 396	FAT 13.1g	SUGAR 15.1g	SAT FAT 3.7g
122	KCAL 457	FAT 13.4g	SUGAR 6.4g	SAT FAT 1.7g
124	KCAL 458	FAT 11.6g	SUGAR 5.3g	SAT FAT 1.3g
126	KCAL 559	FAT 19.5g	SUGAR 8.8g	SAT FAT 3.4g
128	KCAL 525	FAT 19.6g	SUGAR 16.6g	SAT FAT 3.6g
130	KCAL 407	FAT 21.0g	SUGAR 17.0g	SAT FAT 4.2g

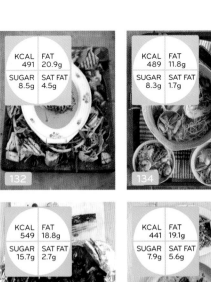

KCAL	FAT
491	20.9g
SUGAR	SAT FAT
8.5g	4.5g

132

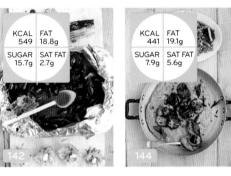

KCAL	FAT
489	11.8g
SUGAR	SAT FAT
8.3g	1.7g

134

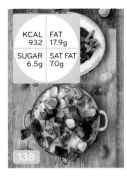

KCAL	FAT
611	21.5g
SUGAR	SAT FAT
15.6g	2.1g

136

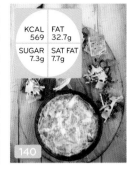

KCAL	FAT
932	17.9g
SUGAR	SAT FAT
6.5g	7.0g

138

KCAL	FAT
569	32.7g
SUGAR	SAT FAT
7.3g	7.7g

140

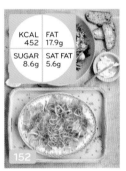

KCAL	FAT
549	18.8g
SUGAR	SAT FAT
15.7g	2.7g

142

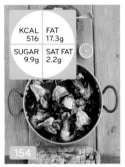

KCAL	FAT
441	19.1g
SUGAR	SAT FAT
7.9g	5.6g

144

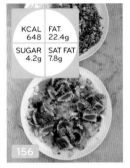

KCAL	FAT
474	14.2g
SUGAR	SAT FAT
7.6g	2.9g

146

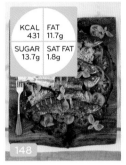

KCAL	FAT
431	11.7g
SUGAR	SAT FAT
13.7g	1.8g

148

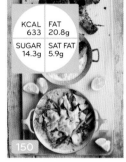

KCAL	FAT
633	20.8g
SUGAR	SAT FAT
14.3g	5.9g

150

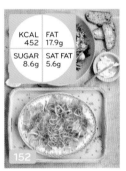

KCAL	FAT
452	17.9g
SUGAR	SAT FAT
8.6g	5.6g

152

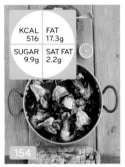

KCAL	FAT
516	17.3g
SUGAR	SAT FAT
9.9g	2.2g

154

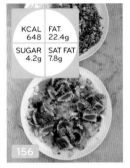

KCAL	FAT
648	22.4g
SUGAR	SAT FAT
4.2g	7.8g

156

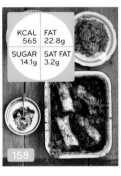

KCAL	FAT
565	22.8g
SUGAR	SAT FAT
14.1g	3.2g

158

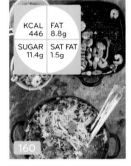

KCAL	FAT
446	8.8g
SUGAR	SAT FAT
11.4g	1.5g

160

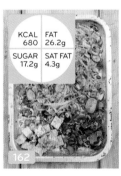

KCAL	FAT
680	26.2g
SUGAR	SAT FAT
17.2g	4.3g

162

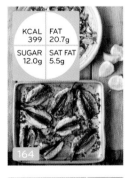

KCAL	FAT
399	20.7g
SUGAR	SAT FAT
12.0g	5.5g

164

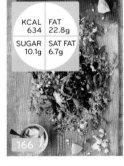

KCAL	FAT
634	22.8g
SUGAR	SAT FAT
10.1g	6.7g

166

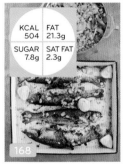

KCAL	FAT
504	21.3g
SUGAR	SAT FAT
7.8g	2.3g

168

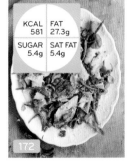

KCAL	FAT
581	27.3g
SUGAR	SAT FAT
5.4g	5.4g

172

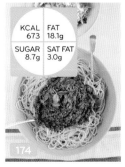

KCAL	FAT
673	18.1g
SUGAR	SAT FAT
8.7g	3.0g

174

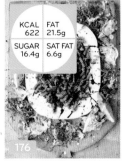

KCAL	FAT
622	21.5g
SUGAR	SAT FAT
16.4g	6.6g

176

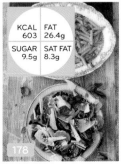

KCAL	FAT
603	26.4g
SUGAR	SAT FAT
9.5g	8.3g

178

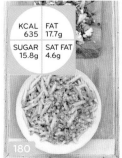

KCAL	FAT
635	17.7g
SUGAR	SAT FAT
15.8g	4.6g

180

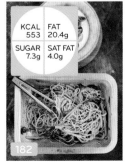

KCAL	FAT
553	20.4g
SUGAR	SAT FAT
7.3g	4.0g

182

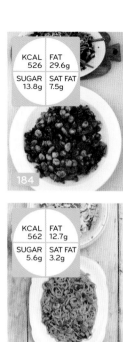

KCAL 526	FAT 29.6g
SUGAR 13.8g	SAT FAT 7.5g

184

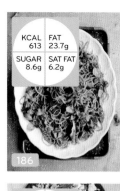

KCAL 613	FAT 23.7g
SUGAR 8.6g	SAT FAT 6.2g

186

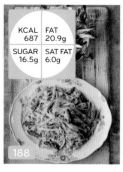

KCAL 687	FAT 20.9g
SUGAR 16.5g	SAT FAT 6.0g

188

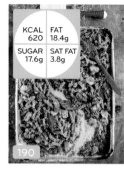

KCAL 620	FAT 18.4g
SUGAR 17.6g	SAT FAT 3.8g

190

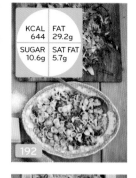

KCAL 644	FAT 29.2g
SUGAR 10.6g	SAT FAT 5.7g

192

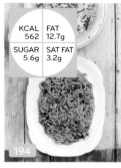

KCAL 562	FAT 12.7g
SUGAR 5.6g	SAT FAT 3.2g

194

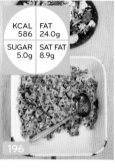

KCAL 586	FAT 24.0g
SUGAR 5.0g	SAT FAT 8.9g

196

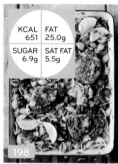

KCAL 651	FAT 25.0g
SUGAR 6.9g	SAT FAT 5.5g

198

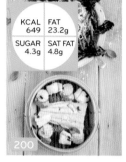

KCAL 649	FAT 23.2g
SUGAR 4.3g	SAT FAT 4.8g

200

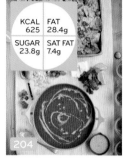

KCAL 625	FAT 28.4g
SUGAR 23.8g	SAT FAT 7.4g

204

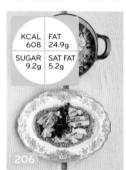

KCAL 608	FAT 24.9g
SUGAR 9.2g	SAT FAT 5.2g

206

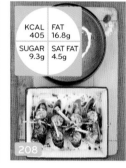

KCAL 405	FAT 16.8g
SUGAR 9.3g	SAT FAT 4.5g

208

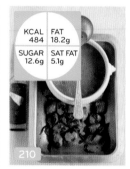

KCAL 484	FAT 18.2g
SUGAR 12.6g	SAT FAT 5.1g

210

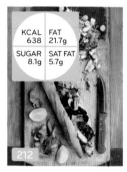

KCAL 638	FAT 21.7g
SUGAR 8.1g	SAT FAT 5.7g

212

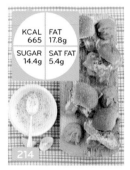

KCAL 665	FAT 17.8g
SUGAR 14.4g	SAT FAT 5.4g

214

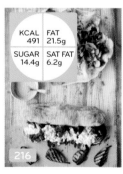

KCAL 491	FAT 21.5g
SUGAR 14.4g	SAT FAT 6.2g

216

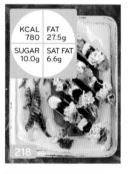

KCAL 780	FAT 27.5g
SUGAR 10.0g	SAT FAT 6.6g

218

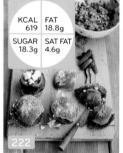

KCAL 619	FAT 18.8g
SUGAR 18.3g	SAT FAT 4.6g

222

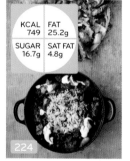

KCAL 749	FAT 25.2g
SUGAR 16.7g	SAT FAT 4.8g

224

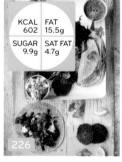

KCAL 602	FAT 15.5g
SUGAR 9.9g	SAT FAT 4.7g

226

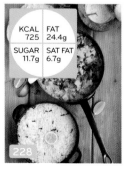

KCAL 725	FAT 24.4g
SUGAR 11.7g	SAT FAT 6.7g

228

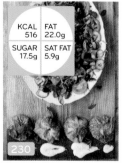

KCAL 516	FAT 22.0g
SUGAR 17.5g	SAT FAT 5.9g

230

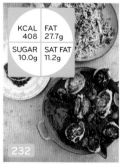

KCAL 408	FAT 27.7g
SUGAR 10.0g	SAT FAT 11.2g

232

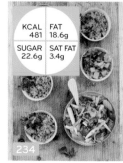

KCAL 481	FAT 18.6g
SUGAR 22.6g	SAT FAT 3.4g

234

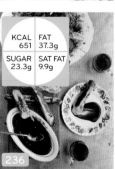

KCAL 651	FAT 37.3g
SUGAR 23.3g	SAT FAT 9.9g

236

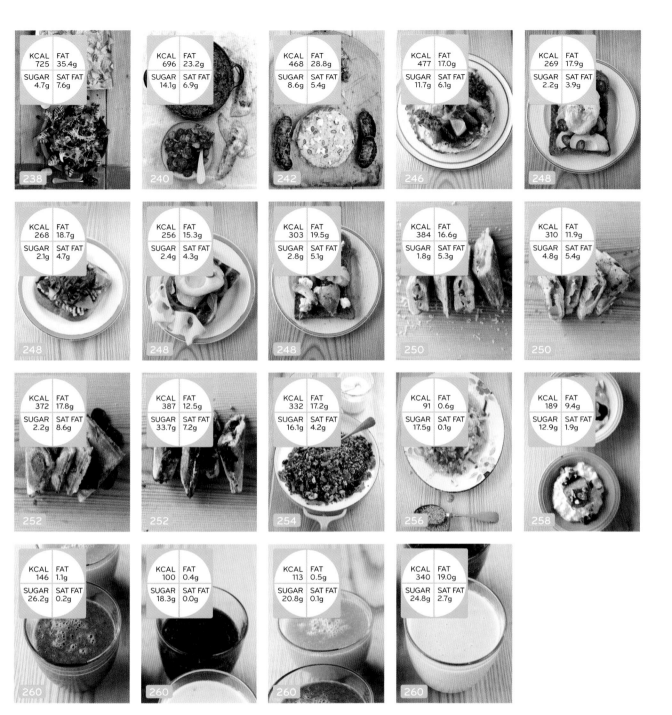

KCAL 725 / FAT 35.4g SUGAR 4.7g / SAT FAT 7.6g 238	KCAL 696 / FAT 23.2g SUGAR 14.1g / SAT FAT 6.9g 240	KCAL 468 / FAT 28.8g SUGAR 8.6g / SAT FAT 5.4g 242	KCAL 477 / FAT 17.0g SUGAR 11.7g / SAT FAT 6.1g 246	KCAL 269 / FAT 17.9g SUGAR 2.2g / SAT FAT 3.9g 248
KCAL 268 / FAT 18.7g SUGAR 2.1g / SAT FAT 4.7g 248	KCAL 256 / FAT 15.3g SUGAR 2.4g / SAT FAT 4.3g 248	KCAL 303 / FAT 19.5g SUGAR 2.8g / SAT FAT 5.1g 248	KCAL 384 / FAT 16.6g SUGAR 1.8g / SAT FAT 5.3g 250	KCAL 310 / FAT 11.9g SUGAR 4.8g / SAT FAT 5.4g 250
KCAL 372 / FAT 17.8g SUGAR 2.2g / SAT FAT 8.6g 252	KCAL 387 / FAT 12.5g SUGAR 33.7g / SAT FAT 7.2g 252	KCAL 332 / FAT 17.2g SUGAR 16.1g / SAT FAT 4.2g 254	KCAL 91 / FAT 0.6g SUGAR 17.5g / SAT FAT 0.1g 256	KCAL 189 / FAT 9.4g SUGAR 12.9g / SAT FAT 1.9g 258
KCAL 146 / FAT 1.1g SUGAR 26.2g / SAT FAT 0.2g 260	KCAL 100 / FAT 0.4g SUGAR 18.3g / SAT FAT 0.0g 260	KCAL 113 / FAT 0.5g SUGAR 20.8g / SAT FAT 0.1g 260	KCAL 340 / FAT 19.0g SUGAR 24.8g / SAT FAT 2.7g 260	

The nutritional information printed in this book is based on theoretical data.
The nutrient values may vary from those published.
Serving sizes are based on recipe recommendations.

Thank you

I want to start by saying a few important thanks to some dear friends who I work with on a regular basis. Most of the people I've chosen to work with on these books have been working with me for a long, long time, although of course there are always a few young whippersnappers coming into the fold! We're a close-knit unit, and whether I'm talking about the talented teams that support me in creating these books, the fantastic personal team that organizes my life, or the dedicated TV crews that make my shows – everything we work on together takes hard work, enthusiasm and energy, which you guys never fail to deliver. So my heartfelt thanks go as follows:

To my dear family, including Gennaro of course, for your continued love and support, thank you.

To David, or Lord Admiral, Loftus – what amazing pictures, brother. As usual you've excelled yourself – lots of love.

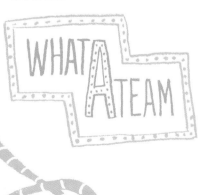

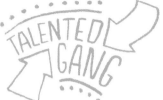

Huge thanks and love to my incredible food team: a wonderful mob of brilliant, talented, massively hard-working cooks, chefs, food stylists, editors and nutritionists. You all make sure everything I dream up actually happens, and your uncompromised commitment to making sure we have the best, most reliable cookbooks is never taken for granted. To the foodies and stylists: mother hen Ginny Rolfe and Sarah 'Tiddles' Tildesley – thank you so much for everything. To my Greek sister Georgie Socratous, bless you and thank you. Christina 'Boochie' MacKenzie, thanks for reining in my swearing, Phillippa Spence, brilliant job pink cheeks, my gorgeous graduate Jodene Jordan, my Brazilian banana Almir Santos and sweet, hardworking Amy Cox – thank you guys. Shout out as well to Barnaby Purdy for his creative energy and Becky Bax for all the help on the shoots. Big love to Abigail 'Scottish' Fawcett for all your brilliant help with recipe testing.

To my cracking food teamers back at the office: Pete Begg ♪ they call it, they call it, they call it, they call it ... AP ♪ and gorgeous ladies Claire Postans, Jo Lord, Helen Martin and Bobby Sebire. You give me amazing support and keep our team on track; I couldn't do it without you. Huge thanks to my nutrition ninjas, who worked closely with me across every recipe in this book: Laura '**** ninja' Parr and Mary Lynch – great job girls.

To my wonderful girls on words: Rebecca 'Rubs' Walker, my NEW editor, thanks for doing an absolutely brilliant job. Thanks as well to the rest of my editorial team, curly/ straight-haired Bethan O'Connor and Malou Herkes. And of course, to Katie Bosher, my EX-editor – thanks for everything as usual. You started this journey with us in London, and helped us finish it from the other side of the world.

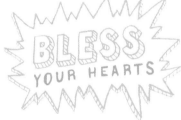

Thanks and love to my lovely publishers at Penguin, who have been just perfect for the last 15 years. You trust me and believe in my instincts, which is amazing. To Tom Weldon, my good friend and the big boss at Penguin, thank you for all your support. To Penguin's brilliant creative director John Hamilton, thank you for all your guidance throughout the books and over the years – still loving it, mate. Thank you to Louise Moore and Lindsey Evans. To the wonderful women on production, Juliette Butler and Janis Barbi – the level of stress and standards you work to are amazing, big big thanks. And to the rest of the cracking team: Tamsin English, Claire Purcell, Jo Wickham, Clare Pollock, Elizabeth Smith, Chantal Noel, Kate Burton, Lucy Beresford-Knox, Nathan Hull, Naomi Fidler, Stuart Anderson and Anna Derkacz – thank you. And finally, to Nick Lowndes and his team of lovely copy-editors, proofreaders and indexers: Annie Lee, Caroline Pretty,

Pat Rush, Shauna Bartlett and Caroline Wilding. Thank you for being so fantastic, diligent, caring, brilliant, clever people, for putting up with my obsessive tweaks, changes and bending of the rules when it comes to the English language, and thank you for working so tightly with my words girls – what a team we have together.

Massive thanks to the lovely girls and guys at Interstate, Jayne Connell, Lucy Self, Christina Beani, Louise Draper, Nigel Gray, Iain Hutchinson, Brian Simpson and Ben Watts. It's always a pleasure working with you, and as per usual I love the beautiful, clean, fresh designs – thanks for helping me make this so good (interstateteam.com).

Thanks also to the gang at Superfantastic, Simon Collins, James Verity and Rachael Ball Risk, who did the cover – great job. It's always fun working with you guys (wearesuperfantastic.com).

Big shout out to my CEO John Jackson, managing director Tara Donovan and my deputy/the matrix/the black widow/the Theydon tongue Louise Holland for all their amazing support. Big thanks to my personal team: Richard Herd, Holly Adams, Amelia Crook, Sy Brighton, Beth Powell and Paul Rutherford. You guys arrange the chaos that is my life and, most importantly, make sure that I have the right amount of time with my family, as well as unadulterated time to concentrate on my books and everything that surrounds them. Thanks as well to Therese McDermott, my PR manager Peter Berry and the lovely Louisa James on marketing for all their help. And to the rest of the guys at my offices, thanks so much for all the hard work you put in daily on my behalf.

And now to the gang at Fresh One Productions . . . half of you lot have been with me a very long time and the other half are freelancers, but all of you are incredibly talented and devoted to whatever project I throw you on. First and foremost, a massive thank you to Zoe Collins, Roy Ackerman and Jo Ralling, who are the heart of Fresh One and genuinely brilliant, talented people. We've built Fresh One together and it's a truly brilliant British independent production company with heart, soul and massively high standards and I'm so proud. Thank you to Nicola Pointer, Mike Matthews and Emily Taylor, the most wonderful, talented series producer, series director and production manager for all their support. To keep up with me and do what you do at the level you do is phenomenal – I really appreciate it and the long hours. Thanks as well to the rest of the brilliant production team: Nicola Georgiou, Gudren Claire, Katie Millard, Nicola Hartley, Shuo Huang, Kathryn Inns, Kirsten Hemingway, Dee Driscoll and Joseph Spiteri-Paris.

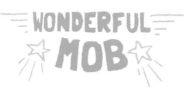

To Luke Cardiff, an amazing cameraman, and gaffer Mike Sarah – you guys have been with me since day one on *The Naked Chef* and I really appreciate every single job I do with you. And to the rest of the fantastic crew and camera team who are super, super talented and top boys, Dave Miller, Jonathan Dennis the jib, Simon Weekes, focus pullers Pete Bateson and Mihalis Margaritis, grip Andy Young, Crispin Larratt and Godfrey Kirby on sound, Paul Casey, Matt Cardiff, Sean Webb, Louise Harris, Steffen Vala and Joe 'son of Mike' Gavshon-Sarah. Shout out to the Timeslice team and their massive camera rig. Big thanks as well to the hard-working edit team: Jen Cockburn, Tony Graynoth, Dan James, Dan Goldthorp, Steve Flatt, Barbara Graham, Joanna Roscoe and James Hart.

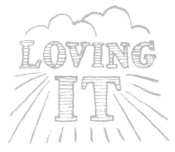

This book has been massively connected with the accompanying TV series so huge thanks to the head of Channel 4, Jay Hunt, and to their daytime commissioner, David Sayer, for being brilliant, trusting me, and letting me get on with it. Thanks to Tim and Sarah Mead and their gang, and Emma Evison, John Artley and the rest of their team for the integration support.

Thank you to Maria Comparetto who keeps me looking presentable on these shoots, and to lovely Julie Akeroyd and Lima O'Donnell. Big shout out of course to the three Gavins and Frank who kept the crew beautifully fed and did an unbelievable job (mobilemouthful.com). And thank you to Zoot & Steve for all your help.

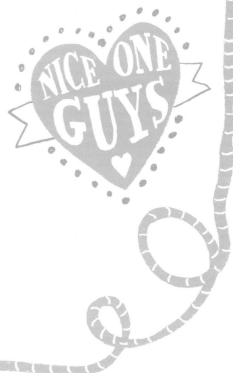

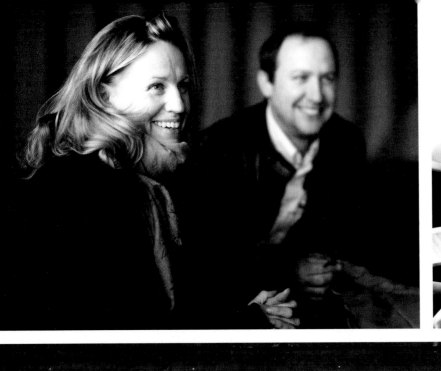
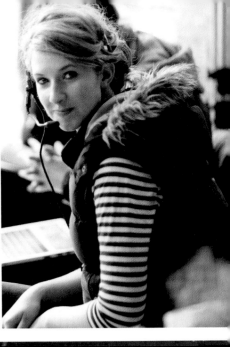
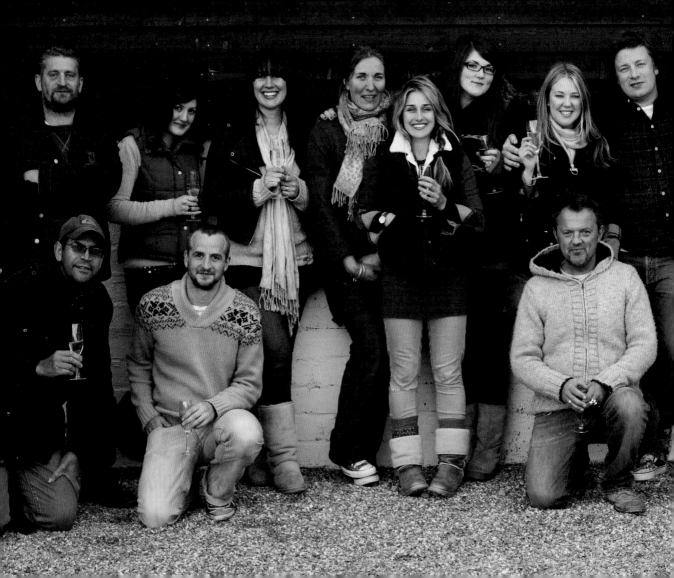

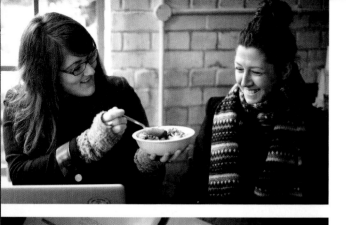

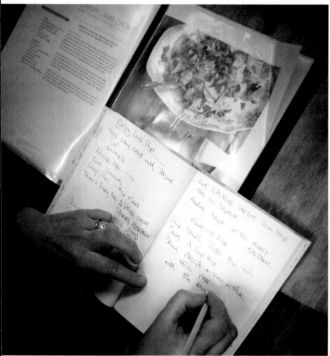

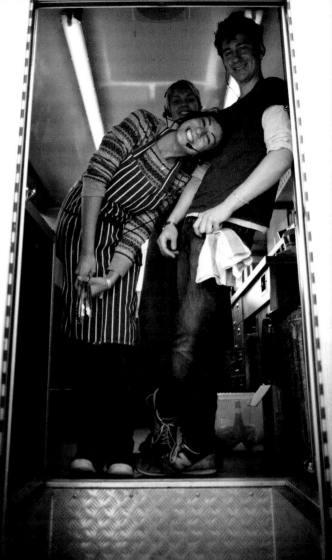

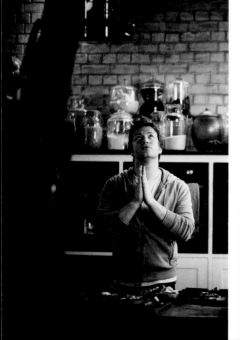

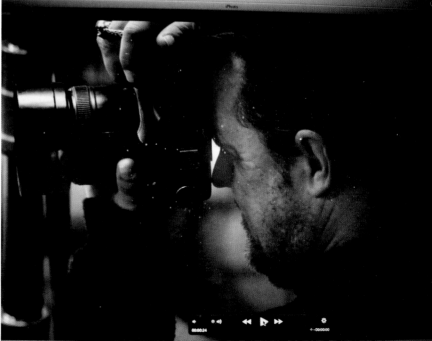

INDEX

Recipes marked v are suitable for vegetarians

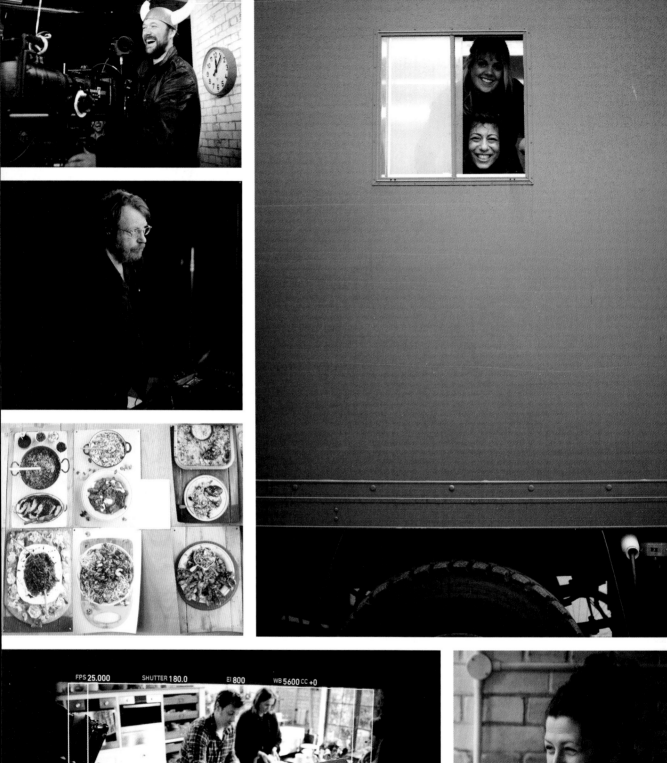
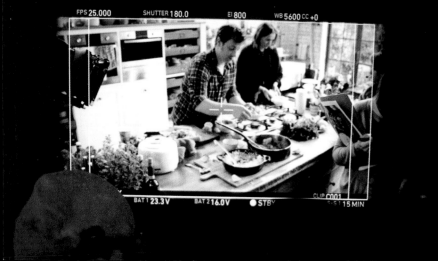
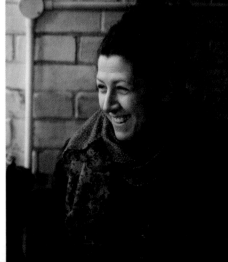

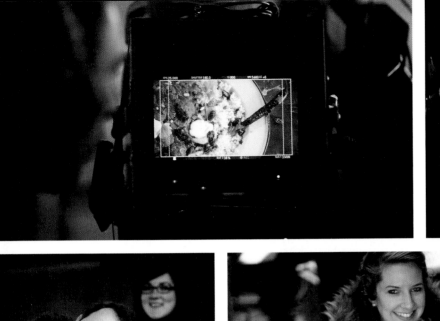
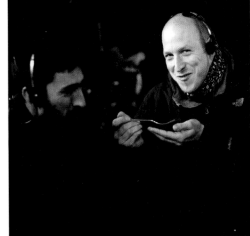
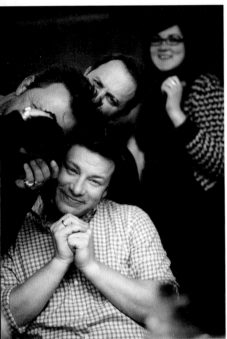
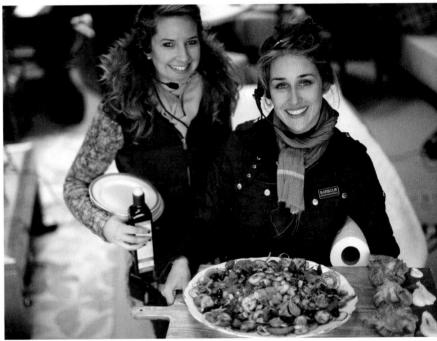
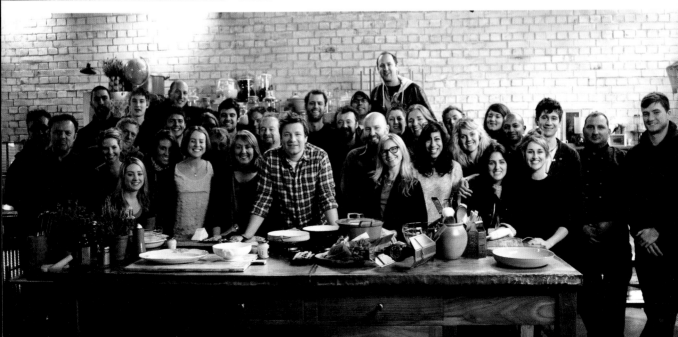

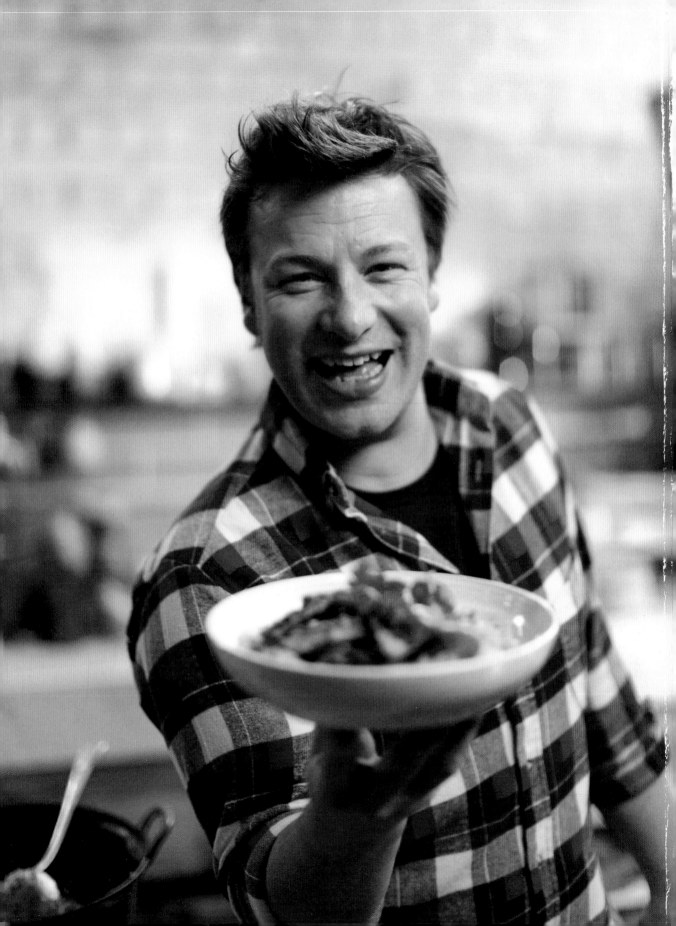